ISBN: 978-0-9994,

Author: Christopher J. Centeno, MD

Medical Illustrator: Christopher J. Centeno, MD

Edited by: Karen Aldridge, RHIA

This book was originally created as an eBook and there are numerous hyperlinks throughout the book.

You can access all of these hyperlinks within the eBook at: http://www.regenexx.com/orthopedics2/

Dedication: To my best friend—my beautiful wife, and to my great kids who put up with me writing this book. They inspire me every day.

Talk to Regenexx

Phone: 855-463-2763
Email : ortho2@regenexx.com
Find a Regenexx doctor near you : Regenexx.com

Contents

Chapter 1: Introduction

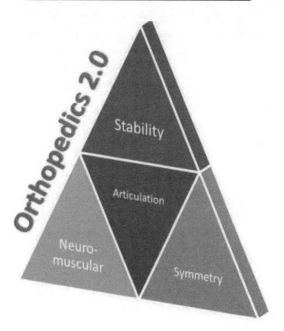

Introduction

First, this book is part of a two-decade quest to find what I have termed the "<u>Unified Field Theory</u>" of the musculoskeletal system. Physicists have long sought a single "theory of everything" that ties together all other theories into one grand explanation of the universe. I've sought to do the same for the musculoskeletal system. Many theories abound about how to diagnose and treat joint, muscle, tendon, ligament, and spinal problems. Orthopedic surgeons have a surgical approach, family-practice and sports- medicine practitioners another conservative approach, chiropractors their own alternative approach, and physical therapists yet another. Within chiropractic, physical therapy, and alternative medicine, there are literally hundreds of wholly different theories about what's wrong with the body and how best to address these problems. Having studied many of these, I always found a kernel of truth and some interconnection between them. As the research in this area has become more robust in the past 20 years, many of these concepts can now be vetted by scientific observation rather than intuitive guesses.

This book contains my own theory of how the musculoskeletal system works and offers a way to organize that information for both doctors and patients. The reader should note that while many of the components of this new theory are supported by rigorous scientific research, the whole package as I present it hasn't been studied using what doctor's call "level-I evidence." This type of medical evidence means that randomized controlled trials have been performed and the treatment approach has been found to be effective. Having said that, most of what we do today for patients with musculoskeletal problems is not supported by level-I evidence. This includes joint arthroscopy, microfracture surgery, labral repairs, all spinal surgeries (including fusion, laminectomy, and discectomy), tenotomy, realignment surgeries (high-tibial osteotomy, lateral releases), rotator cuff repair, ligament repairs, arthroscopic and surgical debridement, chiropractic adjustments, acupuncture, massage, and most all physical therapy. These surgical and nonsurgical approaches all lack the type of rigorous scientific support (level-I evidence) that shows they are effective. In fact, when some of these procedures have been studied in controlled trials, they have often been shown to be no better than placebo surgery or no surgery. (Arthroscopic knee debridement is the most recent procedure shown to have no benefit.)

This is an Internet book that instead of being about one hundred pages long is really several thousand pages long. How is that accomplished? The science behind many of these concepts would create an unwieldy publication that would be too difficult for patients to read and follow. By publishing this book on the Internet, I can easily hyperlink to scientific abstracts and other references so the reader can delve deeper into any subject or simply read the basic explanations. In addition, my goal is to allow patients to submit questions and feedback so the book can be updated and improved. To submit questions or ask for clarification on any part of this book, send an e-mail to the author by clicking here.

What is Orthopedics 2.0? In particular, Orthopedics 2.0 doesn't refer to the discipline of orthopedic surgery or its successor. While orthopedic surgery may well be used as a part of Orthopedics 2.0, Orthopedics 2.0 has a bigger focus beyond just fixing one part of the musculoskeletal system (bones, joints, muscles, tendons, and ligaments). We focus on each part of the neuromuscular system as it is interconnected to the whole and as it is articulately formed together through alignment and stability.

While the focus of this book is nonsurgical, there will always be situations where the best approach is surgical. What will likely occur over the next one to two decades is a slow and steady movement toward less-invasive orthopedic-type procedures—what we call *interventional orthopedics*. This is identical to what's occurred in other areas of medicine, such as cardiology, which now has fewer more-invasive open-heart surgeries and more X-ray–guided catheter procedures.

Interventional orthopedics represents the shift from joint salvage to repair. When the focus shifts to repair, the amount the physician needs to know increases exponentially. The pyramid at the beginning of the introduction outlines what our clinic uses to evaluate the musculoskeletal system. While I use stem cells in daily practice, it's important to note that helping patients is often not as simple as injecting magic stem cells. This book details the system our clinic uses to decide which procedures and therapies to apply as well as the way we look at joints, muscles, nerves, bones, tendons, and ligaments.

The problem with repairing the musculoskeletal system is its complexity. Think about your car. You know there are critical components necessary to keep it running. The wheels have to be aligned or the car won't go straight and the tires will wear unevenly. The connections between the wheels, axle, drive shaft, and engine have to be flexible and allow fluid movement. The engine, as it turns the drive shaft, has to be well oiled. As the engine cranks up to even faster speeds, the connections had better be stable or the whole thing will fly apart. Finally, your engine has miles of wiring and small computers on board to monitor the whole thing and to regulate the activity of the engine, brakes, gasoline usage, and monitoring systems.

Now think about your body and its bones, joints, muscles, tendons, ligaments, and nerves. The same principles of alignment, good joint connections, stability, and sound wiring (nerves and minicomputers that impact everything from the timing of muscle firing to the information about joint position) apply. Regrettably, our surgical approach, to date, has too often just focused on bringing the car into the shop to replace a few worn parts or shave them down so they fit a little better, but it has not considered how the parts got that way. Let's look at that analogy now as it applies to a person.

If a 40- or 50-something-year-old patient who runs every day is suddenly diagnosed with right-knee arthritis, shouldn't we ask ourselves why only the right knee was impacted? Could it be that for years the right knee was getting worn down due to poor alignment? We'd all accept this premise at face value; a misaligned front wheel and axle could cause the right front tire to wear faster than the left. Yet, for some reason, our medical-care system often ignores why one joint wore out faster. The reason: if the plan is to replace the joint, who cares?

But what if we wanted to save the joint? Would it matter more? Absolutely! This is the reason for the Ortho 2.0 approach and this book. When the shift is moved from replacement to repair, it matters how the joint got that way, if the joint is stable, if the surrounding muscles are firing correctly to protect the joint, whether the alignment is correct to support a healthy joint, and if the wiring is in order.

While stem cells are a great advance and represent a cutting-edge tool, their use without considering all of these other things doesn't get patients where they want to be, which is having a joint they can count on for many years to come. In this book, we'll look at all of the parts of the Orthopedics

2.0 paradigm listed above or, as my partner coined the term, **SANS**. This stands for **s**tability, **a**rticulation, **n**euromuscular, and **s**ymmetry. *Sans* in Latin means "without"; hence, the focus of this book is to leave you sans pain.

Our History in This Field

Our website makes the bold claim that we invented orthopedic stem cell therapy. In fact, that's true. I and my partner, John Schultz, began using stem cells to treat orthopedic issues, like knee arthritis, shoulder rotator cuff tears, and low-back disc issues back in 2005, before anyone else. It was years before there was even another provider interested. Hence, we've learned a lot about what works and what doesn't.

I became interested in stem cells in 2004, when a paper was published that showed that you could regenerate a damaged low back disc in a rabbit by injecting stem cells. We began our first injections using both a same-day stem cell isolation as well as culture-expanded stem cells grown in the lab to get more cells. This was a two-year IRB-approved study where we charged nothing. While our patients with joint arthritis did well, it took another one to two years beyond that to figure out how to use stem cells and other things to effectively treat the spine.

So, everyone in this space who is using stem cells to treat orthopedic injuries learned from someone who learned from someone who learned from someone who learned from us. Regrettably, like a bad game of telephone, this means that most clinics that are offering this kind of care don't know what they don't know.

Interventional Orthopedics in Action

Before we get started looking at the SANS system in more detail, let's first take a look at a new movement in medicine that builds off of it— interventional orthopedics. This approach is different from traditional surgical orthopedics. However, as you review these advances, realize that what I'm describing here are advanced procedures that only a handful of physicians across the United States can pull off. Meaning, a nurse in a chiropractor's office or your local orthopedic surgeon won't have the experience and training to perform these procedures.

So let's look at some of those differences.

Joint Replacement vs. Stem Cells: The surgical approach is to amputate the joint and insert an artificial joint. What are the risks of cutting out a joint? A dramatic rise in <u>heart attack</u> and <u>stroke risk,</u> <u>wear particles from the joint prosthesis,</u> and <u>toxic metal levels in the</u> <u>bloodstream</u>.

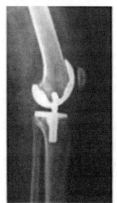

The interventional approach? <u>Many joints with arthritis</u> <u>are unstable,</u> so the physician places injections in the ligaments that need to be tightened to produce a more stable and better functioning joint. With a high degree of skill, using guidance, the stem cells are then placed into the portions of the joint that need help. Can this work? <u>Our treatment registry data suggests that it</u> <u>helps many patients. We have also conducted a</u> <u>randomized controlled trial that shows the same thing.</u>

Rotator Cuff Tears: The surgical approach is to sew the tear and hope it heals. However, too often it doesn't heal—with <u>rates of surgical failure as high as 6 in 10</u>. In addition, <u>big tears fare even more poorly</u>. Why? Many rotator cuff muscles and tendons tear because they have <u>poor blood supply</u> and <u>fewer stem cells,</u> leading to weak tissue. In addition, all too often, the extensive bracing required causes the rotator cuff muscle to atrophy, making it even weaker still.

The interventional approach? Precisely inject platelets or stem cells

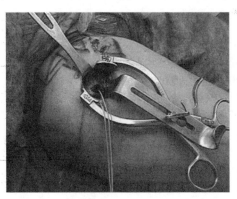

under ultrasound guidance to prompt repair by improving the blood supply and the strength of the tissue. Since often no brace will be needed, atrophy of the muscles in less likely. <u>In many patients</u> <u>with rotator cuff tears</u> <u>treated this way, our</u> <u>registry data shows very</u> <u>promising results</u>. Our early randomized controlled trial data also shows the same.

Anterior Cruciate Ligament (ACL) Tears: The surgical approach is to remove a torn ACL and install a copy. The <u>problem is that the fake ligament goes in at too steep an angle and isn't able to stabilize the knee like the original equipment</u>. Because of all of this, <u>retear rates are very high with athletes being six times more likely to retear the same or the opposite ACL.</u>

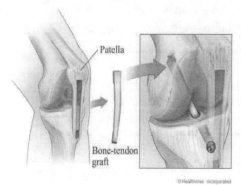

Patella

Bone-tendon graft

© Healthwise, Incorporated

This is likely because the new ligament has none of the same fine-tuning position sensors of the original. Finally, <u>the rehab time until full play can be six months to a year.</u>

<u>The interventional approach</u>? Use the MRI image to map the location of the tear, and then use real-time X-ray to place a needle into the tear. Place stem cells into the tear to heal the area. The rehab time to full activity can be as little as a few weeks to two to three months.

Low-Back Disc Bulge: The surgical approach is to cut out the bulge that's pressing on a spinal nerve causing sciatica. The problem? Discs don't heal. <u>Cutting out the bulge is like sanding down a bump on a bike tire, weakening the outer rubber covering and making it more likely to fail.</u>

The interventional approach? <u>Inject platelet growth factors into the area to improve the blood supply around the disc and reduce the swelling</u>. If this doesn't work, <u>inject specially prepared and cultured stem cells into the disc bulge using a novel device to strengthen the weakened and bulged disc.</u>

Ankle Ligament Tears: The surgical approach to chronically loose ankle ligaments is to remove those ligaments and try to reroute tendons through holes drilled into bone to stabilize the area. The downside? For starters, the tendons will never have the same ability to protect the joint as the native ligaments. In addition, the tendons harvested to replace the ligaments all have a function—there are no spare parts in the body. As a result, the area where the tendons were harvested will never be biomechanically the same.

The interventional approach? Locate the stretched areas using active ultrasound imaging with a stress exam (to place the ligaments under stretch). 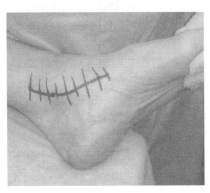 Platelets or stem cells (depending on the extent of the tears) are then placed using exacting ultrasound guidance into the tears in hopes of healing the weak spots. Unlike the long rehab spent on crutches and in a boot using the surgical approach, most interventional patients can go back to activities quickly.

Ulnar Collateral Ligament (UCL) Tears: The surgical approach to this ligament in the elbow that is often injured in throwing athletes, such as pitchers, is "Tommy John" surgery where the ligament is replaced with a tendon. Many athletes' careers end here; however, some go on to play a few more years after losing one to two seasons.

The interventional approach? Use ultrasound stress testing to diagnose areas of weakness often missed on an MRI. Then place platelets or stem cells into these exact spots. Because this is only an injection, recovery is quicker and players return sooner.

Knee Meniscus Tears: The orthopedic surgery approach to a partial meniscectomy is to remove parts of a torn meniscus to try and relieve pain. However, is removing parts of an important shock- absorbing structure a good idea? Several studies show more arthritis for patients who get parts of the meniscus removed. In fact, several recent studies have shown that for patients with arthritis and a meniscus tear, it's often doubtful that the meniscus tear seen on MRI is causing the pain. For patients with that problem, if they have surgery on the tear, the results are no better than just getting physical therapy. Finally, even if the patient is younger and has no arthritis, recent research shows that <u>meniscus surgery is no better than a fake procedure</u>. The most common orthopedic surgery in the United States is partial meniscectomy.

The interventional approach? First, treat any lax ligaments that may

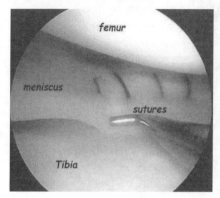

have also been injured but are often overlooked. Next, carefully map the location of the tears using ultrasound imaging, and <u>inject platelets or stem cells (depending on the severity of the tears) into these specific sites</u>. Recovery is quicker because no surgery is done and nothing is removed.

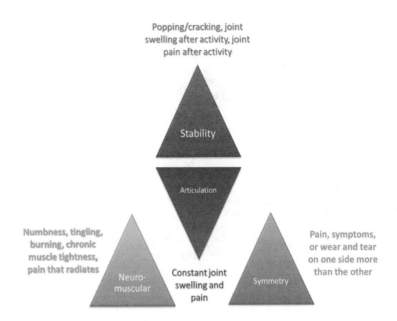

This book is designed so that if you read the next few pages, you'll have gist of the message. The book is also rich in infographics—diagrams that allow you to use pictures and text to better understand the content. Finally, the pages that follow this section describe the concepts in more detail.

So, if you're really busy, start here and end here for now. Read the rest later.

The SANS concept breaks your pain problem into its root causes in four areas: stability, articulation (joint), neuromuscular, and symmetry. (See next page.)

If you have chronic pain of almost any type, from arthritis to spine pain, you will be forever at its mercy if you don't understand its four parts. If you understand these, however, you can take control. So, pay attention!

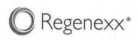

STABILITY
The ability of a joint to tightly move as it was designed without extra motions that might hurt the joint.

ARTICULATION
The health of the joints. Shock-absorbing tissues like cartilage; spacer tissue such as meniscus; or stabilizing tissues such as labrum can be damaged.

S A
SANS
TREATMENT APPROACH
N S

www.regenexx.com

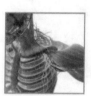

NEUROMUSCULAR
The nerves drive the muscles. Nerves that are irritated or compressed cause pain and may be less able to promote muscles to properly fire.

SYMMETRY
The left/right and front/back balance of the body. When the body is asymmetrical, certain parts get injured or wear out faster.

Stability: Your joints and spine may have small amounts of extra motion that is literally slowly destroying them. The real shocker is that many highly trained physicians and surgeons will likely never tell you about this instability. More concerning is that it can generally be fixed with a few simple injections or exercises.

Stability means a joint that moves with the surfaces in general alignment, all the time. Ligaments are the living "duct tape" that prevents the joint from catastrophic failure. You also need them to make sure the joint doesn't give too much when you stress it hard. Examples include when you walk fast, run, cut (the rapid lateral moves common in sports and exercise), or lift weights. On the other hand, muscles provide the slight adjustments that keep the joint surfaces in very precise alignment as you move. The muscles fire in a symphony of movement with millisecond timing and micrometer precision to make all of this happen. How do you know if you have a problem with instability? You may or may not feel your joint popping and cracking—this tends to happen when the instability is severe. You may have pain or swelling after activity. If you don't feel these things, your joint may be more stable, but it may have more subtle problems that lead to a more rapid progression of arthritis.

Articulation: This is a fancy word for joint. Your joints allow

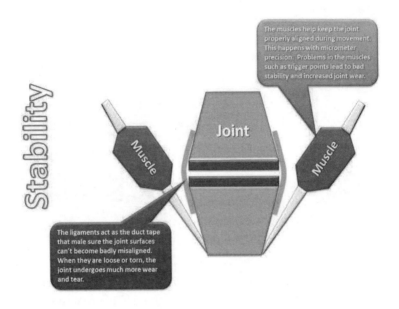

movement in very specific ways. Your hip has a different pattern of possible motion than your shoulder, which is still different from your ankle. A joint is generally made of two bones that come together that are cushioned by cartilage and by a spacer or guiding tissue (for example, a meniscus or a labrum). A joint is also surrounded by a tough leathery covering called a joint capsule and is further reinforced by ligaments. If you want to stay active as you age, you need to learn more about the status of your joints as healthy joints are required for maximum activity.

Everything you do injures your joints a little bit. The million-dollar question is whether they're able to keep up and repair the damage. Stem cells live in all of our joints and are like little repairmen. As we age, there are less of these repairmen, so at some point, wear and tear can exceed the ability of the joint to repair itself and arthritis begins. Many physicians have begun to supplement this repair capability using various technologies, including stem cells.

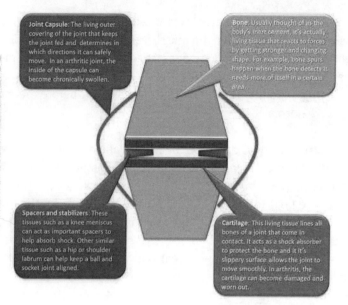

Neuromuscular: Your nerves drive your muscles, yet this fact seems lost on much of medicine today. We'd all accept that when the nerves are severed, muscles die (think Christopher Reeve's spinal cord injury that led to his severe muscle atrophy). Yet what happens when smaller amounts of nerve irritation are present? If you have a chronically tight or weak muscle in your arm or leg, you might not

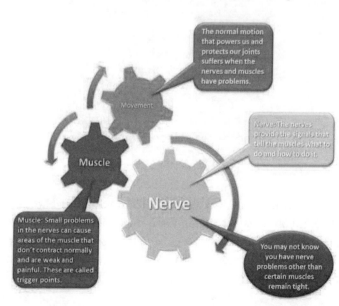

think it's due to an irritated nerve, especially one in your neck or back, but it may be. When the muscles are impacted, they develop tight and weak knots known as trigger points. All the muscle strengthening in the world won't help a muscle when it has lots of these trigger points. They need to be cleaned out before the muscle can work normally.

Symmetry: Why does one knee get arthritis and not the other? Why is the arthritis in one hip or shoulder worse? Sometimes these things are due to prior injury and sometimes to lack of symmetry. Our bodies are built to work well only when each side is exactly like the other. When one of our joints loses normal motion, you can bet other parts will be impacted. When one leg is shorter or one ankle turns in more, again certain parts will wear out faster. Given how important left/right and front/back symmetry is, it's amazing more attention isn't paid to the problem. In order to get well, you must try to reestablish normal symmetry.

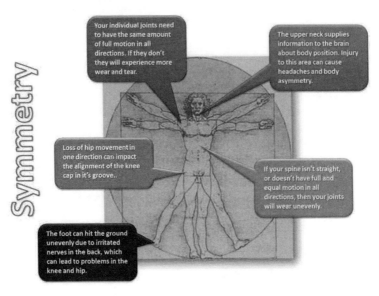

In order to understand why you have chronic pain and how best to get rid of it, you must understand and deal with all issues in the SANS system. You must address any instability issues, problems with your joints, and irritated nerves and muscle trigger points, and, finally, get your body as symmetrical as possible. This book will explain how the

Orthopedics 2.0 approach and the Regenexx procedures can help address these issues.

Summarizing the State of the Field I Helped Create

As discussed, I was the first provider on earth to perform many of these stem cell procedures to help orthopedic problems, so I'm one of the few "fathers" of this field. However, while there are a few good physicians out there trying to do good work, there has also been an explosion of out-of-control hype and poor care. Hence, before you get into the meat of this book, this statement-and-response section covers some things to look out for.

I went to a "stem cell therapy" seminar put on by a local chiropractic office, and they claimed they could regrow new cartilage in my "bone on bone" knees. They even showed me before and after X-rays and told me that my stem cells were too old, so they use stem cells taken from birth tissue.

First, no stem cell therapy in existence will regrow large amounts of new cartilage in a "bone on bone" knee. However, that's not to say that a real stem cell therapy may not help reduce pain and increase function. In addition, there are no living and functional stem cells in the commercially available birth-tissue products used by these clinics. Hence, the claims of this seminar were a scam.

- Chiropractors, acupuncturists, and other providers who show you before and after X-rays of knees that appear to show increased joint-space width are involved in imaging tricks; let me show you how this is done.

- The birth-tissue products these clinics use have no living stem cells.

- State attorney general offices are onto and are prosecuting the chiropractors involved in these hype-driven "stem cell" scams.

The interesting thing is that these products do contain growth factors, like platelet rich plasma. So, in the right kind of problems, they can help pain. However, in "bone on bone" arthritis, they will generally only provide a couple of months or relief.

A local orthopedic surgeon or pain doctor uses a system called "Lipogems" and offers "fat stem cell therapy."

Lipogems is a system that produces a fat graft, but it is not a stem cell therapy in that there are no, or very few, free stem cells dislodged by this processing. While this therapy may or may not help your knee pain or other issue, if it's being advertised as a "stem cell therapy," that's hype. Now, I've been told by patients asking these questions online that their orthopedic surgeon is well respected and is the team doctor for the [insert name of sports team here]. However, all orthopedic surgeons in practice today have had the same amount of stem cell basic biology training in medical school or residency, which is *none*. Meaning that in our experience, most don't know what they don't know.

A doctor told me he gets stem cells from my blood.

This is also a scam. There is no significant stem cell population in your blood. This ruse is often used by doctors who don't feel like learning how to perform a bone marrow aspiration to access stem cells. Having said that, your blood has platelets, and concentrating them by creating platelet-rich plasma can help certain types of orthopedic problems.

Some doctor told me all I needed was a magic infusion of stem cells and I would be fixed.

How is that supposed to work? How will the cells infused into your veins get to the injured spot? Are these even the right kind of stem cells?

See these quick links:

Stem cells injected into your veins will end up in your lungs, not in your knees.

Fat stem cells aren't as good at helping orthopedic problems.

A doctor says that he uses "exosomes" and these are better than stem cells.

Think of an exosome as a guided missile. Stem cells can "fire" exosomes at other cells, and these little packets contain information that give the other cell instructions. Thus, stem cells use exosomes as a communication method to help orchestrate the complex dance of tissue repair.

However, some providers have begun taking the media in which stem cells are cultured (which contains exosomes) and using this rather than the cells. While this may have some use in helping tissues heal, it's a bit like using a guided missile where the guidance system has been removed. Meaning the stem cell is the intelligence behind which missiles to fire at what cells with which instructions and when. Take away the stem cells and you go from smart missiles to dumb bombs.

More Common Concerns...

I have pain in my joint(s), and my doctor said it's due to arthritis.

How did your joint get this way? It didn't just happen by itself. Was it an injury? Why can someone else get the same injury and not get arthritis? Can you slow down arthritis? Why does someone get it in the first place? Is there something you can do to prevent other joints from getting it?

See these quick links:

- Knee surgery for arthritis doesn't work. What can I do to preserve cartilage?

- Why your ACL ligament may be loose and you don't know it...

I have a torn or frayed ligament, tendon, meniscus, or labrum.

If the tear was due to an injury, why did just that tendon tear? If not an injury, what caused the tear? Why didn't it heal? Can I prevent other structures from tearing? Can it be fixed without surgery? Is surgery even a good idea?

See these quick links:

- <u>Is a knee meniscus tear causing my pain, or does everyone my age have meniscus tears</u>?

- <u>Why operating on a hip labrum tear may be a really dumb idea</u>.

I have pain in my head, neck, upper back, or lower back/hip.

There are many things that may be causing your pain outside of a slipped or bulging disc. The gold standard of figuring out which structure is causing pain is imaging numbing injections. Did you know that there may be abnormalities on your MRI that were missed?

See these quick links:

- <u>Diagnostic blocks may save your spine from a useless surgery</u>.
- <u>What nobody ever told you was wrong with your MRI.</u>

Chapter 2: Stability

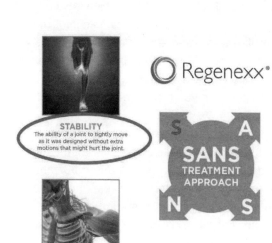

STABILITY
The ability of a joint to tightly move as it was designed without extra motions that might hurt the joint.

ARTICULATION
The health of the joints. Shock-absorbing tissues like cartilage; spacer tissue such as meniscus; or stabilizing tissues such as labrum can be damaged.

NEUROMUSCULAR
The nerves drive the muscles. Nerves that are irritated or compressed cause pain and may be less able to promote muscles to properly fire.

www.regenexx.com

SYMMETRY
The left/right and front/back balance of the body. When the body is asymmetrical, certain parts get injured or wear out faster.

Regenexx®

S   A
SANS
TREATMENT
APPROACH
N   S

"In all of Shakespeare's plays, no matter what tragic events occur, no matter what rises and falls, we return to stability in the end."

Charlton Heston

Take this 3-question quiz to see if this section applies to you. If you answer any question with a yes, you may have a stability problem.

1. The area I'm concerned about gets very sore or swollen after I exercise. Y N
2. I hear cracking/popping in this area when I do certain activities. Y N
3. This area often feels like it's loose or moves too much. Y N

Stability

What does it mean to be stable? Stable in a mechanical sense means resistance to falling apart or falling down. For your body, joint stability is a very big deal, yet you likely haven't been told the whole story. You see, you've only been told about a very unstable joint that requires surgery to fix a completely torn and retracted ligament. Yet it's the instability you don't know about that's **slowly frying** your joints, one movement at a time. Discovering which joints have this kind of instability, called subfailure, may save you from a joint replacement.

What is subfailure instability, and how do I know if I have it? *Subfailure instability* means that the surfaces of the joint aren't kept in exact proper alignment during movement. Why is this important? When the joint surfaces uncontrollably crash into one another or even just can't be kept in perfect alignment, the joint wears down much faster. An unstable joint literally experiences many times the wear and tear of a stable joint, and bone spurs form. Since stability in many joints is the number one determinant of whether that joint will have a long happy life or become "old" before it's time, it's a wonder more time isn't spent assessing this component of joint health.

Let's slice and dice joint stability a little further by separating the type you've heard of and that is usually easily diagnosed from the type that will slowly destroy your joints and will likely never get diagnosed. There are two major types of instability: surgical and subfailure.

Surgical instability is less common than its more prevalent cousin—subfailure instability. However, surgical subfailure is usually the only type that the orthopedic establishment treats. This means that a joint (either a peripheral joint, like the knee, or a spinal joint) is very unstable and unable to hold itself together at all. In these cases, surgery is often needed to stabilize the joint. Examples would be a completely torn and retracted ACL in the knee or severely damaged ligaments in the spine where a spinal cord injury is feared if the spine isn't surgically stabilized. A surgically unstable knee may need a new cadaver or artificial ACL implanted through surgery, while a surgically unstable spine may need a fusion where the bones (vertebrae) are fused together with additional bone. Regrettably, neither is a perfect solution as the <u>new ACL will go in at the wrong angle</u> and the fusion will <u>cause other spinal segments above and below to be overloaded</u>.

Subfailure means that the ligament *hasn't* completely failed (torn apart like a rubber band), but instead it's only partially torn, degenerated, or just loose. This much more common type of instability often doesn't require surgery and is characterized by small extra motions in the joint just beyond the normal range. In fact, if you have this type of instability, *you likely aren't aware you have this problem.*

Our understanding of subfailure instability is younger and more immature, so while we have some diagnostic tests to detect this type of instability, our understanding of what is normal and abnormal is only now coming into focus. However, this type of instability is quite real, and it's a clear and long-term insidious drag on joint health. <u>A good example of this is the research showing that replacing an ACL in the knee will lead to earlier and more significant arthritis in that knee joint.</u> Why? While surgeons take great care to make sure the replaced ligament is identical to the torn one, <u>there is no way to ensure the replacement ACL has exactly the same specs as the original.</u> The new ligament can be too tight or too loose or may simply not have the identical load-bearing characteristics of the original equipment.

More on Subfailure: It's All About Your Ligaments and Your Muscles

There are two types of subfailure instability: ligament and muscular. Passive ligament stability keeps our joints from getting badly misaligned. Think of ligaments as the living duct tape that holds our joints together. An example would be an ACL in the knee, which keeps the tibia bone from sliding forward under the femur bone. Without this ligament, every step would cause the joint to experience a potentially damaging shift. On the other hand, active muscular stability is made up of the firing of muscles that helps keep the joint aligned as we move and represents the stability fine-tuning system. Our joints tend to want to slip slightly out of alignment as they bend, twist, or slide, even with intact ligaments. As this happens, signals are sent to selective muscles that surround the joint so that they adjust and correct the alignment. Without this active system, our joints (especially ones like the shoulder that are dramatically dependent on muscle stability) would be "sloppy." This muscle firing is a muscular symphony, with microsecond precision being the difference between beautiful joint music and an asynchronous chorus of potentially damaging "joint noise."

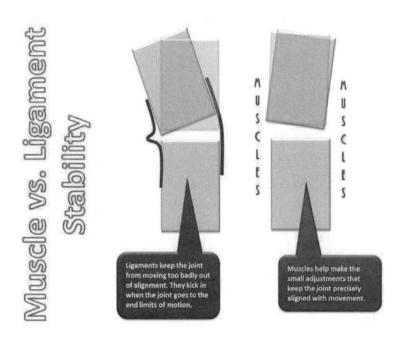

Ligaments keep the joint from moving too badly out of alignment. They kick in when the joint goes to the end limits of motion.

Muscles help make the small adjustments that keep the joint precisely aligned with movement.

Let's start with your finger. Move it back and forth right now. As you move it only a little bit, there isn't much resistance to motion. If you move it a lot (bend it all the way back), there's more resistance to motion. In fact, it eventually stops. This is because the ligaments that surround the joint (along with the covering of the joint, called the joint capsule) prevent this excessive motion and ultimately stop the joint from moving. This is what happens in a functioning joint-stability system—the passive elements (ligaments) keep the joint surfaces from getting badly aligned.

So, what do the muscles do again? The muscles provide the fine tuning. They act as constant stabilizers for the joint, keeping it in good alignment while we move. This small area where the joint must stay to prevent damage as we move is called the "neutral zone."

So, in summary, stability is about both muscles and ligaments. Our muscles provide constant input to the joint to keep the joint alignment fine-tuned as we move. When the joint moves too much, the ligaments act as the last defense to prevent joint damage from excessive motion. Think for a second about what would happen if the muscles didn't work in microsecond precision to keep your joints perfectly aligned? What would happen if the ligaments didn't check excessive motion when the joint went a little too far? Both of these things are recipes for sudden disaster or for slowly damaging the joint one movement at a time!

Now let's explore how poor stability may be harming your joints. We'll start first with the backbone of your skeletal system, the spine. If this important structure isn't stable, nothing else will be quite right. We'll then move out to instability in joints, like the shoulder and knee.

The Spine Is a Marvel of Stability Engineering

The spine is advanced engineering. The spinal column is made from a series of blocks that stack one upon the other and provide a base of support for the extremities and protect the spinal cord and nerve roots. These interlocking blocks (vertebrae) use the same stability model as described above—muscles and ligaments. This same system also applies to all of your joints, like the knee, shoulder, hip, elbow, and ankle.

Now let's look at how the spine stays stable. What happens when you place a bunch of blocks one on top of the other? This tower of blocks gets less stable as the pile gets higher (see left). One way to stabilize this high tower of blocks would

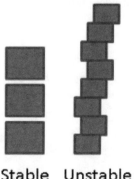

Taped blocks-
Stable, but
immobile

Stable   Unstable

be to tape the blocks together. This would make the blocks more stable but wouldn't allow much motion. You could use more rubbery and flexible tape than duct tape or Scotch tape, but again you'd either end up providing too little stability (highly elastic rubbery tape that gives a lot when you stretch it) or too much (duct tape or Scotch tape that's more rigid).

Imagine if we had to move all of the taped blocks so they could bend into a C-shaped curve (see right)? How stable would your blocks be then? The right kind of tape (ligament) would likely allow this motion, but the individual blocks would still start to shift against each other. This shifting could result in disaster, as the spinal cord runs through a hole (spinal canal) inside the blocks, and the spinal nerves exit between the blocks through a special bony doorway (foramen). As a result, too much movement between the blocks means nerve damage or worse, a spinal cord injury. This is the dilemma of the spine: how to stack lots of blocks (about 25 high in most people) while keeping the whole thing stable and flexible and at the same time protecting the nerves. Is there a solution? Yes, **the muscles** provide that solution. They keep the blocks (vertebrae) aligned against one another with millimeter precision while you

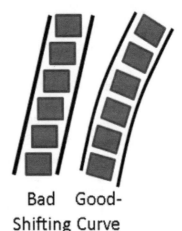

Bad   Good-Shifting Curve

bend and twist. In fact, since the muscles are so important for a healthy spine, it's unsettling that most physicians couldn't tell you which group of muscles provides this stability.

Are there specific ligaments that live in the spine? Look at the picture below where I have highlighted in red all of the ligaments that are visible from the back view of the spine and pelvis. There are ligaments everywhere! Wouldn't you think these ligaments might be a target for therapy? Has any surgeon ever said that your ligaments were normal or abnormal? Regrettably, our medical care system, outside of a few exceptions, ignores the ligaments that act as the duct tape to hold your body together!

Spine Ligaments to Get to Know

I have shown the low-back ligaments, but many of these are the same in the neck and upper back.

Supraspinous/Interspinous Ligaments: The "duct tape" that runs down the very back of your spine in the middle, on top of, and between the spinous processes. These are the bony bumps you can feel in the middle of the spine in the back (thinner people will feel more of them). They control the motion of the vertebrae when you bend forward. They are commonly injured in car crashes and other trauma and may become degenerative with age.

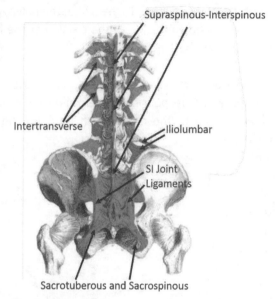

Labels: Supraspinous-Interspinous; Intertransverse; Iliolumbar; SI Joint Ligaments; Sacrotuberous and Sacrospinous

Intertransverse Ligaments: These go between the bony processes (transverse processes) that stick out of the side of the spine. They control motion in the vertebrae when you bend to the side. If bending that way makes things worse, these ligaments may be stretched.

Iliolumbar Ligaments: These go from the side of the L5 and sometimes L4 (bottom low-back vertebrae) to the side of the hip/pelvis area. They are major stabilizing ligaments of the most mobile part of the low back. Problems in these ligaments can refer pain down to the thigh and front of hip. To learn more, <u>click here</u>.

Sacroiliac (SI) Joint Ligaments: These are the massive ligaments at the back of the sacroiliac joints (the joints between the tailbone and back of the pelvis/hip). Women have more issues here than men, and these can be stretched during childbirth, falls onto the butt, and trauma. The pain is often in this area at the back of the hip and can refer down the leg.

Sacrotuberous and Sacrospinous Ligaments: These ligaments anchor the bottom of the tailbone to the rest of the pelvis, and when injured, can refer pain down the leg to the outside of the foot, almost like a pinched S1 low- back nerve.

Alar and Transverse Ligaments: Alar and transverse ligaments in the upper neck are responsible for holding your head on. The alar ligaments (blue to the right) reach up from the C2 vertebra and attach strongly to the skull, while the transverse ligaments (red to the right) hold the pivot point of the C2 vertebra tightly to the C1 bone, allowing you to turn your head without getting a spinal cord injury. These ligaments can be injured in car crashes or injuries where something hits the head. Their laxity can cause everything from dizziness to visual changes to severe headaches.

Skull Fits Here

Occipital Bone (Base of Skull)

C1

Alar Ligament (right)

Accessory Ligament (left)

Atlas C1

Capsule of Atlantoaxial Joint

C2

Deeper Part of Tectorial Membrane

Transverse Ligament of Atlas

Axis (C2)

Upper Cervical Spine: Posterior to Anterior View with Ligaments

Muscular Stability in the Spine

If muscles help solve the problem of keeping the blocks aligned against each other while the spine moves, which muscles are these?

For most of the spine, this special muscle is called <u>multifidus</u>. These small muscles travel from vertebra to vertebra to keep the spine bones in proper position. <u>In the 1990s, some very smart scientists noted that these muscles were smaller than usual in most patients with chronic low-back pain</u>. Since that time, <u>atrophy</u> (when the muscles get smaller and weaker) of these and other spinal muscles is a known cause of low-back and leg pain. These muscles can be seen on almost all MRIs, and <u>numerous research articles have correlated shrinkage of these muscles with back or leg pain</u>, but, regrettably, this atrophy is almost never commented on in radiology reports!

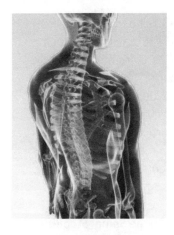

If this muscle is such a big deal, why haven't you ever heard about it, and why has nobody told you that it's a problem? Good question! Regrettably, the vast majority of medical providers, physical therapists, and chiropractors haven't read about this research. Why? The multifidus hasn't had a champion to take it from the pages of medical journals to the prime time of major medical conferences. This is despite the fact that to make sure your spine bones stay aligned and aren't constantly bumping into spinal nerves, these muscles have got to be firing on all cylinders all the time.

What Happens When the Muscular Stability System Goes Down?

Remember that ligaments are only one-half of the joint stability equation—muscles are the rest of the equation. When the muscles fail to align the joint, the joint becomes sloppy. Too much movement is allowed in all the wrong directions. This causes excessive wear and tear on the joint (<u>arthritis</u>), whether the joint

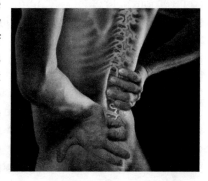

is a disc in the low back or a knee, shoulder, ankle, or hand joint. Obviously, the first way to help this problem would be to strengthen muscles around the joint. However, just getting the stability muscles stronger sometimes isn't enough. **Sometimes the nerves telling the muscles what to do don't work well.** In my experience, patients who have this issue don't know they have it. In cases like this, no amount of strengthening will help until the nerve issue is addressed (see the "Neuromuscular" chapter).

The Heavy Head: A Weak and Compromised Spinal Stability System

Many patients who have been in a car crash tell us that their head feels heavy. How is this possible? The head is a bowling ball being balanced on the end of a stick (the spine). There are muscles at the top of the neck as well as in the front and back. These deep muscles help to hold the bowling ball on the stick. As you'll see in the section on symmetry, losing the natural curve in the neck can push the bowling ball forward on the stick. In addition, the articulation section will discuss how injuries to the neck joints can take the stabilizing muscles off-line. All of this can conspire to make someone feel like they have a bowling ball instead of a head!

A Dramatic Example of What Happens When the Spinal Stability System Is Off-Line

A number of years ago, I went for a several-hour mountain bike ride. I had just read a research paper that discussed how factory workers showed weaker back stabilizing muscles after being in a bent-forward posture for several hours. Regrettably, that day my own back would become an example of this phenomenon. Right after the ride, I went to pick up my son, felt a pop in my back, and collapsed. It took days to recover, and for the first 48 hours, I was in agony. In my case, the lumbar multifidus was "off-line" from being bent forward on my bike, which caused irritation of the nerves. This led to a period of instability in that spinal segment, a time during which I was more likely to get injured. Essentially, that spinal segment was left completely unprotected by the spinal muscles when I went to pick up my son. My back, thus, went down in flames like the Hindenburg! This "multifidus" off-line mechanism, whether it's caused by bike riding or just something else that irritates nerves, is believed to be the cause for most acute back pain episodes.

I've felt the same thing occur a few more times, most notably once while dead-lifting weights in the morning (after sleeping in a flexed posture all night). These are all dramatic examples of what happens when stabilizing muscles are turned off. How do I get these muscles back online and almost immediately fix my pain rather than lying in bed for days? An epidural injection around the nerves reduces the nerve swelling and generally turns these important muscles back on. Usually, after one of these low- back meltdowns, I can exercise on a limited basis within hours of getting an epidural. However, as you'll learn later in this book, all epidurals aren't created equal.

Fusing the Spine or Any Joint: Usually a Bad Idea

This past decade has seen an explosion in the number of fusion surgeries. What does this mean? The concept is simple. If some joint is unstable, you just bolt it together and put bone in the area so the joint becomes immobile solid bone. Is this a good idea? Think about the fact that your body is a finely tuned machine where millimeters of extra or lack of motion can cause problems. Now think about what would happen if I made a joint not move at all. It wouldn't be long before the joints above and below would begin to wear out from the extra pressure, as after all, the forces have to go somewhere.

The most common fusion surgeries are in the spine, ankle, and wrist. Spinal fusion surgeries are associated with a myriad of complications and problems. In addition, as you might imagine, the joints and discs above and below the surgical site that's fused get fried very quickly. This means a patient can spend a lifetime chasing the next level as it degenerates faster because of the fusion. While I have seen a handful of patients in my career who really need and would benefit from spinal fusion, these patients, in my opinion, represent only about 5% of all of the patients who are currently being fused in the United States. In fact, regrettably, treating the chronic pain suffered by spinal fusion patients could keep a pain management doctor in any community busy full time.

Another common area that gets fused is the ankle. <u>This is called a</u> <u>"triple arthrodesis" for the three joints that must be fused.</u> In reality, <u>an X-ray of the ankle of these patients looks like they had a bad trip</u> <u>to the hardware store.</u> This procedure is often used to treat ankle arthritis. Like spine fusion, it just causes arthritis above and below the fusion site, usually making the patient worse in the long run. In addition, since the ankle joint doesn't move, impacting how the patient walks, other issues in the knee, hip, and spine can develop. The wrist, a very complex series of bones that move precisely against each other to allow normal hand function, can also be fused. All of the same issues as discussed above apply. In addition, hand function is obviously compromised.

Stability in Joints

Your joints are tuned to submillimeter (hair width) precision. They move in certain ways that are generally defined by the ligaments that hold them together. If you want some idea of how complex these ligaments are, just look at the directions of all of the ligament fibers around the human hip (see right), each one coursing a certain way to allow just enough motion in just the right direction—no more and no less.

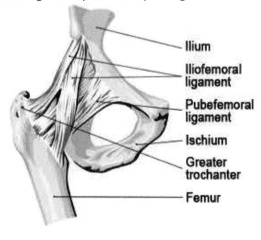

- Ilium
- Iliofemoral ligament
- Pubefemoral ligament
- Ischium
- Greater trochanter
- Femur

In addition, the muscles around joints also act as a secondary, but no less important, stability system. Probably the joint most reliant on muscular stability is the <u>shoulder</u>. The <u>shallow socket of the shoulder</u> means the <u>ball of the humerus</u> has lots of opportunity to get out of place. The <u>rotator cuff muscles</u> help to keep the ball in the center of this shallow socket. Other joints rely on similar control mechanisms. Some joints have more intrinsic stability because they have deep sockets (<u>like the hip</u>) or are tightly bound by ligaments (<u>like the knee</u>). However, the goal of the muscles crossing the joint is the same—to keep it aligned while the joint moves. Despite different designs, all joints from your elbows to your toes are dependent on muscles to fine-tune their alignment.

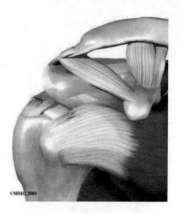

The Lip around the Socket: Labrum Surgery Mania

Both the shoulder and the hip have an additional stabilizing structure called the labrum. This is literally the lip around the socket of the ball-and-socket joint. It does all sorts of important things from adding some additional stability to adjusting muscle tightness and activation to providing cells that can help it repair itself and the cartilage underlying it.

The labrum can be torn, and it has been the target of an explosion in orthopedic surgery this past decade. However, these are very big surgeries with sometimes less than stellar results. For example, one study showed that only about <u>4 in 10 patients thought shoulder labrum surgery was very successful</u>. Other studies have shown that almost <u>7 in 10 patients without hip pain had labral tears on MRI</u>! The interventional orthopedics approach to labral tears is the first to confirm that they're causing symptoms. If they are a problem, then they can usually be <u>treated via precisely targeted injections of platelets or stem cells</u>.

Ligaments That Support Your Joints: What You Don't Know May Be Hurting You

Our modern surgically based orthopedic care system has evolved to generally only treat complete ruptures of ligaments. This is when the ligament breaks and snaps back into pieces. So what happens when the ligaments are just loose? While this is a big problem that can lead to arthritis, this is almost never detected by physicians. Why? The patients with this type of ligament issue aren't surgical candidates. However, once these ligaments can be tightened or helped via simple injections, the lax ligaments become a big target for therapy. The reason is simple: if a loose ligament is frying a joint, why not try to help the ligament? In fact, in many ways, fixing the ligaments would be the foundation for any treatment of the joint, just like fixing the shaky foundation of a house would be the first step before trying to renovate the building.

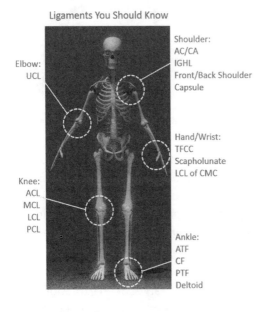

Ligaments You Should Know

Elbow:
UCL

Shoulder:
AC/CA
IGHL
Front/Back Shoulder
Capsule

Hand/Wrist:
TFCC
Scapholunate
LCL of CMC

Knee:
ACL
MCL
LCL
PCL

Ankle:
ATF
CF
PTF
Deltoid

To the left is an overview of the ligaments in your body you should know. Obviously, focus on the areas where you have problems.

Shoulder

• Acromioclavicular/Coracoacromial (AC/CA): These go between the collarbone and from projections of the shoulder blade and stabilize the top/front of the shoulder. These are the ligaments that get stretched in a "separated" shoulder. When loose, they can lead to arthritis in the AC joint, bone spurs that press on the rotator cuff, and degenerative rotator cuff tears.

• Inferior Glenohumeral Ligament (IGHL): This ligament lives at the bottom of the main shoulder joint and keeps the ball from slipping downward, relative to the shallow socket, when you lift your arm above your head. When lax, this ligament can lead to more arthritis in the big shoulder joint as well as bone spurs on the bottom of the joint.

• Front/Back Shoulder Capsule: These ligaments are really just thickenings of the covering of the big shoulder joint that are all tightly bound with the rotator cuff muscles that surround the joint. They keep the ball of the big shoulder joint from slipping too far forward or backward in its shallow socket. If your shoulder has ever been dislocated at any time in your life, it was these ligaments that were likely lax. When these ligaments are loose, we see more arthritis in the main shoulder joint as well as labral tears (the labrum is the lip of the shallow socket).

Elbow

• Ulnar Collateral Ligament (UCL): This ligament is commonly injured in throwing athletes, such as pitchers, or in injuries that involve bending or torqueing the elbow. It's the "duct tape" on the inside of the elbow, and laxity here will lead to arthritis in the elbow joint and pain/swelling after activity. The ulnar nerve ("funny bone") can also get irritated leading to numbness in the little finger side of the hand. There are also other main elbow ligaments on the outside of the joint and around the radius (the bone that allows your hand to turn palm up or down).

Hand/Wrist

• Triangular Fibrocartilage Complex (TFCC): This is the most important ligament you've never heard of. Don't let the long name scare you. It's really just a cushioning and stabilizing system of ligaments for
the outside of the wrist that allows you to use that opposable thumb that separates primates who can grasp things from the lower animals. It can be injured by landing on a hand or thumb or just get degenerative with age or wear and tear. It makes the outside wrist bones unstable and can lead to wrist arthritis.

• Scapholunate Ligament: This is one of many ligaments that holds the many little bones in the wrist together. It is more on the thumb side, and when torn can cause cracking and popping in the wrist and a feeling that the bones are shifting too much. It's usually injured when falling on a hand that's hyperextended.

• Lateral Collateral Ligament of the Carpometacarpal (LCL of CMC): This is the outside ligament of the wrist/thumb joint, the one that gets what's been called "blackberry thumb" or "texting thumb." This ligament usually gets loose with wear and tear and allows the thumb bone to slide out at the base of the wrist, leading to bone spurs. It is also associated with an irritated median nerve (i.e., aka carpal tunnel syndrome).

• There are other wrist, thumb, and finger ligaments, but they are too many to list.

Knee

• Anterior Cruciate Ligament (ACL): The important front-back stabilizer in the middle of the knee joint. This ligament is often lax but rarely gets noticed because it's not the type of "torn in half" injury that needs surgical removal and replacement. When it's loose, it leads to more wear-and-tear-type arthritis.

• Medial Collateral Ligament (MCL): This is an often-injured inside-of-the-knee ligament. Injuries occur when someone is tackled from the side, such as by a football player or a dog. It takes a long time to heal, and in our experience, even after it stops hurting, it's still lax. When it's lax, it can cause the inside meniscus (shock absorber) to move in and out of the joint resulting in wear-and-tear damage to the meniscus. This can cause pain on the inside of the knee.

• Lateral Collateral Ligament (LCL): This is the ligament on the outside of the knee that's linked into complex ligaments that go from the outside of the hip to below the knee. As a result, patients with lax LCLs often feel pain from the outside of the hip to below the knee. When it's lax, it can also cause the outside meniscus to be yanked in and out of the joint, leading to wear-and-tear damage to the lateral meniscus.

• Posterior Cruciate Ligament (PCL): This is the ligament on the inside of the knee that prevents it from being overextended. When it's damaged, the knee can extend too much and the structures in the front of the knee can get pinched (like the front parts of the meniscus). This laxity again often goes unnoticed by physicians.

• Anterior Lateral Ligament (ALL): This is a newly discovered ligament that is on the outside-front of the knee and is often injured when the ACL is torn or injured. It helps to stabilize the knee in rotation and is one reason many researchers think that knee ACL replacement surgeries may be unsuccessful.

Ankle

• Anterior Talofibular (ATF), Calcaneofibular (CF), and Posterior Talofibular (PTF): These are ligaments on the outside of the ankle. They are commonly injured when you "turn your ankle" and are the most commonly stretched ligaments. If you've sprained your ankle and it intermittently gives you problems, these ligaments are likely loose. If they continue to not protect the ankle, then ankle arthritis may already be or may soon be in your future.

• Deltoid: These ligaments are on the inside of the ankle, and when they become lax, they allow too much pronation of the ankle. These ligaments are less commonly injured, but since the tarsal tunnel with its tibial nerve is on the same side, it can also become irritated. When these ligaments are lax, the outside of the main ankle joint (lateral talar dome) can get cartilage lesions.

Microinstability: A Constant Drag on Joint Health

It's important to note that most subfailure instability might not be felt by you as the joint giving too much in the wrong direction—in fact, smaller movements may be happening without your knowledge. These small amounts of extra motion are called microinstability and while any one or ten events might not lead to injury, they can have a big impact as thousands of small insults add up over long periods of time. Even an extra millimeter of motion, when repeated 10,000 times, can damage a joint. As a result, often the best way to look for these small amounts of extra motion is by having a good physical exam by a physician trained to look for these small amounts of extra motion. The American Association of Orthopaedic Medicine is a good place to find such physicians. This group provides educational seminars for doctors

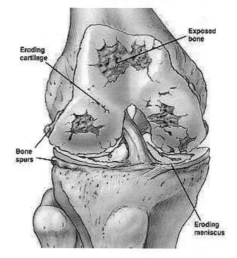

interested in treating instability with injection therapy.

An Example of the Kind of Ligament Damage That Can Be Treated with a Needle

There are three types of damaged ligaments: partial tears, complete nonretracted tears, and complete retracted tears. The best way to conceptualize these tears is by using a big rubber band. Our piece of stretchy rubber can have small tears within it or a tear that doesn't go all the way through. In a ligament, these would be examples of partial tears. Next up in severity is a complete tear where the rubber band is badly mangled in one area and there are small tears that go all the way through the structure, but the band still holds itself together. In a ligament, this is called a complete nonretracted tear as our band hasn't snapped back into two halves. Finally, there is a complete tear where the two halves snap back. In ligaments, this is called a complete retracted tear.

Now consider the ACL as an example. The ACL is a major stabilizer of the knee, and tears of the ligament are common sports injuries. The ACL can have a partial tear where only some fibers are broken but much of the ligament remains intact. It can also have a complete tear without retraction (an area of light color on the MRI, but the ligament hasn't snapped back like a rubber band). Finally, it can have a complete tear with retraction where the ligament fails completely and does snap back like a rubber band. In our clinical experience, a partial tear, a complete nonretracted tear, and even a tear with a small amount of retraction can generally be treated   by placing stem cells into the tear under very precise X-ray guidance. A complete retracted tear requires surgery. Despite this, we still see many patients getting their ACLs surgically ripped out and replaced with an inferior ligament. To learn more about how we treat torn

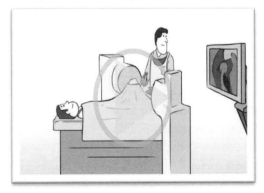

ligaments, like the ACL, with stem cells, click on the video link to the right.

Why Physical Therapy Sometimes Fails

The past one to two decades of supervising rehab programs for patients has taught me that while strengthening the muscles often helps the muscular stability of the joint, sometimes it fails. Why? **The muscles are controlled by nerves**. While much of traditional medicine has focused on big problems in nerves that can be picked up on static imaging, like <u>MRI</u>, or on electrical tests, like an <u>EMG</u> (electromyogram—a test where needles are inserted into the muscles), the more recent research shows that a lot can go wrong with nerves that is generally invisible to these tests. This smaller amount of spinal nerve-root irritation can wreak havoc with the muscles by shutting parts of them down. This problem, despite the research, largely is ignored by physicians. This is because our medical care system isn't yet focused on detecting these smoldering nerve issues.

When a part of a muscle gets shut down by nerves, it may not be responsive to strength training. These shut-down muscle areas are called <u>trigger points</u>. An easy way to get rid of these tight and weak areas of the muscle is trigger point massage, or direct pressure on the area. When this fails, a trigger point injection or dry needling of the spot (<u>IMS or intramuscular stimulation</u>) is often the answer. In our experience, this can allow that part of the muscle to work again and start helping the joint to stabilize. This concept is discussed further in the <u>"Neuromuscular" chapter</u>.

I can't emphasize enough that if traditional physical therapy fails, you must look at whether you have nerve and muscle problems. You may believe that you have no spinal nerve problems, but it's more likely than not that you do and just don't know it!

Why Can't Strong Muscles Substitute for a Bad Ligament Stability System?

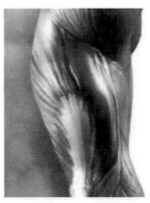

If your joint has one or more loose ligaments, maybe you can just get stronger by doing lots of physical therapy and that will suffice. After all, can't the muscles just substitute for the loose ligaments? As discussed, there are two types of stability systems, the fine-tuning is provided by the muscles while the ligaments prevent serious abnormal joint movements that can lead to catastrophic joint damage. If the ligaments are stretched out a little bit, but still intact, the muscles may be able to substitute and protect the joint in most situations. However, if the ligaments are stretched or damaged so that they allow bigger abnormal motions in the joint, **no amount** of muscular stability will help. In the end, while having stronger stability muscles may help reduce some of the wear and tear, the joint will still get into abnormal alignments that will lead to accumulated damage. So if ligaments are stretched, it's best to tighten them (this can often be done without surgery—see the section on regenerative medicine), and if they're completely torn and retracted, the only option may be to surgically replace the ligament.

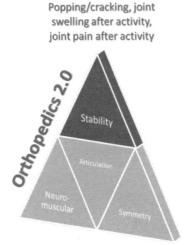

Popping/cracking, joint swelling after activity, joint pain after activity

How Do I Know if I Have a Stability Problem and What Can I Do to Help It?

How do you know if you have a stability problem? Patients often complain of popping or cracking in the spine or joints. They may at times feel sudden shifts in the spine or affected joint. For example, when performing cutting exercises, they may feel their knee "give way." In the neck, patients may feel that by the afternoon or evening they have a "heavy head." In other patients, there may be no perceptible sense of instability or popping/cracking in the joint, just joint pain or swelling after activity. These patients usually have smaller amounts of microinstability.

Regenexx Simple Muscular Stability Tests

When you get evaluated using the SANS system, these are the quick and simple physical exam tests that will determine if you have good or poor stability. There are also other things that will be evaluated, like the status of your spinal stabilizing muscles on MRI. **If you have pain with any of these movements, make sure that you pay attention to the rest of these chapters.**

We expect our patients to be participants in their own recovery, so we want them to take this test on a monthly basis when being treated. If you're a Regenexx patient, before your first evaluation, please take the test, print out the work sheet, and bring it to your first evaluation. If you were given a physical book, you can find the work sheet in Appendix A. If you're not a patient, you can take the test and use the work sheet to record where you are at any given time (click here for a printer friendly link to the work sheet).

Caution! These tests may cause injury or exacerbate the conditions of patients who have a more fragile stability system or who are at a lower level in their stability. Please do not attempt these if you get injured easily. If you do decide to perform this assessment, if you get significant pain during any given test, stop immediately. You are performing these tests at your own risk.

Getting Ready: For some of these tests, you'll need an assistant. You'll also need a timer or clock/watch with a second hand (there are good stopwatch programs on most smartphones).

Neck—Upper Cervical (Scalenes): The first test is simple. Just lift your arms out to your sides and all the way above your head. Is this easy or hard? Can you easily get your arms up all the way? Now have

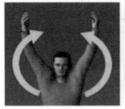
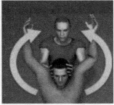

Lift arms above head all the way. Then have someone hold head firmly and retest. Fail if it's easier to lift the arms with head hold.

someone stand behind you and hold your head very firmly. Your head shouldn't move at all as you perform the same hands-over-head maneuver. Was it easier to lift your arms with your head stabilized by someone? If you found it hard to lift your arms over your head without someone stabilizing your head, then you may have upper cervical instability. This means that the muscles or ligaments stabilizing your upper neck may not be strong enough.

If you experience significant pain with this maneuver, stop!

Scoring: If you feel no difference with or without the head hold, then give yourself a 3 here. If you feel a noticeable difference and can get your arms all the way up, you score a 2 If you feel a difference and get your arms over your shoulders but not all the way up, you score a 1. If you can't get your arms over shoulder height, give yourself a 0.

Neck–Deep Neck Flexors: The second neck test was developed by an Australian researcher and is a bit more challenging. Lie on a flat and firm surface, like the floor, and have someone time and monitor you. First, tuck your chin fully and then lift your head 2-3 inches. Have your monitor start the timer. The clock stops when you lose any degree of the chin tuck or your head is unable to maintain the same height. Normal for men is 38 seconds and for women is 29 seconds. If

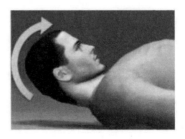

Tuck chin and lift head about 2-3 inches and time. If any loss of height or chin tuck occurs, then stop timing. Normal is 38 sec for men and 29 sec for women.

you can't do this, your deep neck flexors are weak and you fail this part of the test. These are underline important muscles that stabilize the front of your neck. When these muscles are weak, patients often report headaches.

If you experience significant pain with this maneuver, stop!

Scoring: Write down your timed score.

Neck—Extensors: The third neck test was developed by a US physical therapist and tests the endurance of the deep and superficial neck muscles that hold your head up. You first lie facedown on a table or firm bed, making sure your chest is stable (you may want to have someone hold you by placing downward pressure on your upper back). You then hold your head perfectly straight with the face parallel to the floor.

You hold this position and time yourself. You should be able to get to 20 seconds without your neck and head bending (as shown in C) or extending (as shown in D). If you went into position C as you fatigued, your superficial neck extensors are weak. These help to hold your head up. If you went into position D, your deep neck extensors are weak, and the superficial extensors are taking over. In both of these instances, patients with weak neck extensor muscles tend to report a heavy head or fatigued neck by the end of the day.

If you experience significant pain with this maneuver, stop!

Scoring: Write down your timed score.

Shoulder—Rotator Cuff: The test for the shoulder focuses on rotator cuff muscle endurance. The arm is held out to the side with the thumb facing down and pointing toward the floor. The arm is then moved down toward the side and back up to shoulder height. You perform this movement in the three planes shown (behind the body, at the body, and in front of the body). Do this slowly.

If you experience significant pain with this maneuver, stop!

You should be able to do these 10 times in each position (30 reps total). You may be fatigued. If you can't get that far without stopping, you need to strengthen the rotator cuff. These muscles help to stabilize the ball of the shoulder joint in its socket.

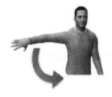

Scoring: If you can get through 30 reps (10 in each plane) without pain (although you may be mildly to moderately fatigued), then give yourself a 3 here. If you can barely do this and

With arm out to the side with the thumb down, move the hand completely down and up in the three planes noted. Pass is at least 10 reps slowly (30 up-down movements).

experience much fatigue and effort or have pain with this test, then you score a 2. If you can't get through all of this due to fatigue or pain you score a 1. If you can't do this at all give yourself a 0.

Core—Abdominals:
There are two stability tests for the lower back, both pioneered by a Japanese researcher. The first is a simple sit-up maneuver where you begin by lying faceup and bringing your hips and knees to a 90-degree position as shown. Make sure you keep your neck

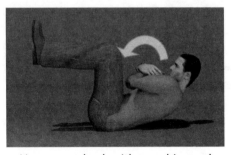

Lie on your back with your hips and knees both at 90 degrees and lift your torso off the ground. Time how long you can hold this position.

flexed. Set a timer and hold this position. The normal time for men are 182 seconds (3 minutes), and for women it's 85 seconds (1.5 minutes).

If you experience significant pain with this maneuver, stop!

If you have a lot of pain with this maneuver, you may have a disc pain issue as flexion places more pressure on the disc.

Scoring: Write down your timed score.

Core—Low-Back Extensors: The next test starts with lying facedown on the floor and placing a firm pillow under your stomach with your hands at your side. The pillow should be firm enough or doubled up so that you can extend your back and lift your chest off the floor as shown. Your neck should remain flexed. Set a timer and hold this position. For

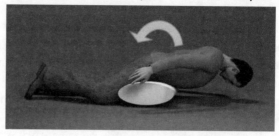

Lie on your stomach on a stiff pillow and extend your back so that your chest is off the floor and hold. Time how long you can hold this position.

men, the normal hold is 208 seconds (3.5 minutes), and for women it's 124 seconds (2 minutes).

If you experience significant pain with this maneuver, stop!If you have pain with extension like this, you may have either a facet or lumbar stenosis problem.

Scoring: Write down your timed score.

Hip/Knee: There is a single test for hip and knee stability as both of these are linked. Here, you stand and then balance on one foot (the side you want to test). You then perform a single-leg squat while trying to keep your body as straight as possible. If you're able to balance so that you're straight for about one-half of the deep knee bend and for the return back up, then you pass the test on that side. If you must tilt your body over to that side and/or

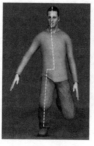
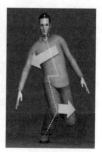

Normal   Abnormal

your knee drives inward, you have poor hip and knee stability and fail the test. If you can't perform the half squat, you fail as well.

Scoring: Write down your timed score for each side as the number of seconds you can hold that side in the position shown in the picture to the left (Normal) versus the right (Abnormal).

Ankle: You can test the ankle from the same standing-on-one-leg position. Count to 10 while balancing on one leg and watch your ankle. With your body straight (which is again measuring your hip stability) and hands to your sides, does the ankle roll or have to move back and forth during that 10 seconds? If so, you have an unstable

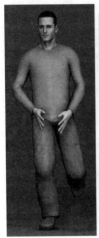
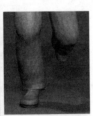
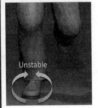

ankle. If not, and the ankle remains rock solid for the 10 seconds, you pass this test. If you have a tough time with this, you may have an ankle stability issue. This can impact things all the way up to the knee and can even, in some patients, cause a kneecap issue.

Scoring: Write down your timed score for each side as the number of seconds you can hold the ankle is stable.

What if I failed some of these tests? This means you have poor stability in these areas. This could be due to pain shutting down muscles, weak muscles, or irritated nerves that make them weaker or misfire. If it's pain, then you have to find and fix the source of that problem. If it's weak muscles, they may just need strengthening. Finally, if its irritated nerves, no amount of getting the muscles stronger will help; you need to reduce the nerve irritation. These things will all be covered later in the book.

As you get treated, use this Regenexx Stability Test as your monthly spot- check to gage your progress. You want to increase your scores in each problem area.

What Other Diagnostic Tests Can Diagnose the Problem and What Therapies Might Help?

Spine Diagnosis:

In the spine, larger amounts of instability can be seen on either low-

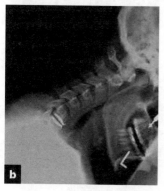

back or neck flexion-extension x-rays. These are tests where the patient looks down and up or bends forward and backward while x-ray films are taken. Regrettably, too often, the technicians that take these films don't push patients far enough into these positions (flexion or forward, extension or backward). If you undergo one of these tests, make sure to push yourself in these motions (without hurting yourself). The research shows that such efforts can reduce the false negative rates of these tests (a false negative is a test that fails to show positive even though the patient has the disease). A newer form of this test is called Digital Motion X-Ray (DMX). This test looks at a moving x-ray view of the spine as the patient is put through various ranges of motion. It can also be used in various peripheral joints, such as the knee, shoulder, and elbow.

Spine Therapies and Exercises

The lowest level of spinal stability training uses ultrasound imaging or other biofeedback devices to help patients contract their multifidus and transversus muscles in the low back. The same type of program can help with neck instability. This program is called deep neck flexor strengthening (strengthens longus colli and longus capitis), and this therapy has research to show its efficacy in helping headaches.

The next level of difficulty for spinal stability is usually where most programs start. If this level of therapy makes things worse, then either it's too advanced for the level of muscle atrophy or there are other issues that have to be addressed (like damaged ligaments, irritated nerves, and painful joints). For the low back, the oldest such program is called dynamic lumbar stability or DLS. In the neck, once patients have mastered lower-level neck strengthening exercises like deep neck flexor strengthening, we have used the BTE multicervical unit, which helps us identify cervical function, physical limitations, and capabilities and allows us to record in real time cervical spine range of motion (ROM) and isometric strength.

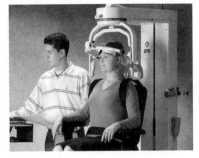

The following link to exercises that help build **core** strength:

Basic   Transversus abdominus
                               Multifidus

Advanced   Spinal Stabilization at levels 1 and 2
                               Spinal Stabilization at levels 3-6 Bosu
Standing Squat

The following link to exercises that provide low-level **cervical** strengthening for severely unstable patients:

Basic   Deep neck flexors level 1
                               Basic Deep-neck flexor level 2
                               Basic Deep-neck flexor level 3
                               Basic Deep-neck flexor level 4

Advanced   Neck and shoulder extensor stability
                               Neck/shoulder stability

Peripheral Joints

For peripheral joints, the most common X-ray tests for stability are for the shoulder AC joint and the ankle. For the shoulder, the x-rays are taken with and without the patient holding weights. For the ankle, the nerves may be anesthetized with a numbing medicine and then the ankle turned, and an x-ray taken at maximum movement.

The goal of both of these tests is to detect too much movement in the joint with stress. As a result, they are often called stress radiographs (another word for X-ray).

For smaller amounts of microinstability (very common), we use various tests. Another method for detecting smaller amounts of instability in the knee is a KT-1000 arthrometer. This is a machine that replicates the physical exam for small amounts of laxity in the ACL ligament. There are also other devices that can test many different joints in a similar fashion. We currently use the Telos Stress Device.

While diagnostic tests for instability and hypomobility are just becoming popular, the best way to diagnose these problems is still through history and exam. An experienced physician can compare joint motion from side to side (good side versus bad side) as well as stress the joint to look for signs of instability. As discussed above, the American Association of Orthopaedic Medicine (AAOM) is a good place to look for doctors experienced in diagnosing smaller amounts of instability. Many orthopedic surgeons can also diagnose instability, but realize their focus will be on the larger amounts of instability that we have called surgical instability. Thus, the focus will often be on surgical solutions.

Peripheral Joints Therapies and Exercises

Shoulder: Rotator cuff exercises can be helpful. They are very commonly prescribed and taught by most physical therapists.

- Rotator cuff exercises
- Shoulder stabilization exercises
- Shoulder strengthening exercises

Knee: Knee stability exercises are also commonly taught in many physical therapy programs. The Kinesio Taping programs (look up McConnell Taping Techniques) are a good bet for kneecap pain and combine taping to provide better proprioceptive feedback from the joint being trained. This method can also be used for other joints.

- Knee stability exercises

Ankle: Rocker boards, BAPS boards, and other unstable platforms can be used by therapists to help the leg muscles provide more efficient stability in the ankle.

- <u>Ankle stability exercises</u>

Stretched ligaments causing unstable joints can often be helped without surgery by <u>prolotherapy</u> or <u>platelet-rich plasma (PRP) injections</u>. This will be discussed further in the next chapter.

Chapter 3: Articulation

STABILITY
The ability of a joint to tightly move as it was designed without extra motions that might hurt the joint.

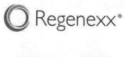

ARTICULATION
The health of the joints. Shock-absorbing tissues like cartilage; spacer tissue such as meniscus; or stabilizing tissues such as labrum can be damaged.

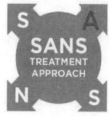

www.regenexx.com

NEUROMUSCULAR
The nerves drive the muscles. Nerves that are irritated or compressed cause pain and may be less able to promote muscles to properly fire.

SYMMETRY
The left/right and front/back balance of the body. When the body is asymmetrical, certain parts get injured or wear out faster.

"The universe as we know it is a joint product of the observer and the observed."

Pierre Teilhard de Chardin

Articulation

Articulation means joint. This could be any joint, like peripheral joints (knee, shoulder, hip, ankle, elbow, wrist, etc...) or the joints between two spine bones (the disc and facet joints). While peripheral joints are generally different from a spine disc, they share more in common than not. Both spinal and peripheral joints allow motion and do so in a controlled manner. A joint has certain standard components.

Cushioning: In the peripheral joints, the cushion is usually the cartilage or meniscus. In the spine, the middle of the disc, called the nucleus pulposus, serves as the cushion. Both of these are not inanimate pieces of rubber, but living tissues with cells and structure. Once these components die off, these joints lose their ability to provide shock absorption.

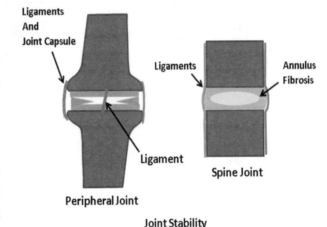

Stability: This is provided by the joint capsule (tough outer covering of the joint) or the ligaments that help hold the joint together. In the disc, this is provided by the tough outer covering and surrounding ligaments. In addition, many joints have another element called a labrum to hold a ball in a socket. These are found in the shoulder and hip.

Notice that while our entire medical care system in orthopedic surgery revolves around joints, in the SANS system, the joint is simply one part of a bigger picture where ligaments, nerves, muscles, and symmetry is equally important or more important. What are the implications of paying too much attention to the joint? Imagine that instead of being focused on the musculoskeletal system, we were concerned about the urinary system, but instead of considering the kidney, ureter, bladder, and urethra, all we focused on was the bladder? This is too often what we do today; we focus on the joint and exclude the rest of the musculoskeletal system.

Arthritis in a joint means that the parts and pieces, like cartilage, meniscus, and bone, are degenerating or wearing down. So how do we access the degree of arthritis in a joint? We image it using an MRI. However, do these images paint an accurate picture of why you hurt?

Imaging Insanity, or the Very Poor Correlations Between Structure and Function

Every patient I have ever met wants an MRI, which is a fancy picture of the soft tissues that's created by powerful magnetic fields. While our practice uses MRIs to help define pathology, what if I told you that if you placed a bet that I could tell from your MRI what was causing your pain, I could give you only 1:1 odds (50/50)? Let's start with the most pervasive musculoskeletal MRI finding of the late 20th century, knee meniscus tears. If your doctor sees a meniscus tear on your MRI, it's a sure thing that the meniscus tear is causing your pain, right? **Wrong**. A study published in the *New England Journal of Medicine* showed that about 60% of patients without a history of active knee pain have meniscus tears on MRI. This study was completed by the famed Framingham Heart Study group. They observed two groups of middle-aged to elderly patients, with one group having recent active knee pain and the other having no recent or remote history of knee pain. Turns out they both had about a 60% rate of having meniscus tears on their MRI. This study calls into question the reasoning behind hundreds of thousands of knee surgeries performed over the past two decades. Since many meniscus tears aren't likely causing the patient's pain, **why are we operating on them?**

How about the findings on hip MRIs—surely these must accurately show the cause of my pain? Not so much. In fact one study showed that many of the findings that surgeons rely upon to make the diagnosis of hip impingement (aka FAI or cam impingement) are found in normal patients without hip pain! In addition, another study

<u>shows</u> that the bone spurs surgeons often remove to reduce impingement are actually protecting the joint from more arthritis. So why are we removing these bone spurs? Why are we performing hip arthroscopy often based on a cursory exam and a hip MRI?

Other studies that have tried to link abnormal MRIs to pain have also been equally disappointing. For example, several low-back studies have shown that patients with severe problems on MRI are often pain free, while other patients with severe pain often have limited structural changes on MRI of the spine. Once we find problems on MRI, our traditional medical care system often likes to operate on that joint. Let's look a bit more at whether that's a good or bad idea.

Which Joint Is Causing the Pain?

Once a joint, tendon, or ligament is seen on MRI to have problems, we still don't know if it's causing the pain. While in joints like the fingers, it's easy to see which one likely is causing the pain, other joints don't lend themselves to an exam.

Take, for example, the hip and the sacroiliac (SI) joint. Both can refer pain to the hip/groin area. It's very hard to get your fingers near the hip joint as it's buried in inches of muscle. As a doctor, you can feel the back of the SI joint, but most of it is buried inside the pelvis. How do you know which one is causing what the patient reports as "hip" pain? The only way to know for sure is to "block" one or the other (inject numbing

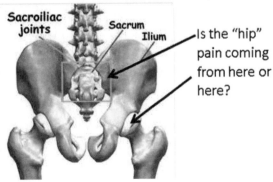

medicine to kill the pain from one). Since the accuracy of the injection is important (meaning if the doctor injects the numbing medicine into the muscles instead of the joint, you're no closer to solving the mystery), fluoroscopy (real-time X-ray imaging) or ultrasound are used to place the medication. There are many other joints where it's difficult to tell which is the "pain generator" (the joint causing the pain). Other examples include the facet joints in the spine, the small joints of the foot and ankle, and the multiple joints of the wrist.

Regrettably, we've seen through the years patients who have been told they need a hip replacement based on a bad hip X-ray. We then block the hip, only to have the patient report minimal pain relief. We then block the SI joint, and the patient gets complete relief of pain. So, the moral of this story is, before considering major surgical procedures, be absolutely sure you know which joint is causing the pain! Replacing a hip that doesn't hurt isn't going to help you much!

One word of caution. Many physicians use an anesthetic known as Marcaine, or bupivacaine, to numb joints for diagnostic purposes because it lasts longer than other anesthetics. However, this anesthetic has been shown to damage cartilage, and the <u>American Academy of Orthopaedic Surgeons has warned their members not to use it</u>. Therefore, you need to ask which numbing medicine will be used. <u>If it's Marcaine, or bupivacaine, ask the doctor to substitute 0.25-0.5% ropivacaine as this has been shown to be more cartilage friendly</u>. However, also realize that this numbing medicine is often only found in maternity wards unless the doctor special orders it, so he or she may have never used it. Lidocaine, or Xylocaine, is another anesthetic that can be used. While it has less cartilage toxicity than Marcaine, it still has some negative effect.

Are There Joints in Your Spine?

Your spine has little joints about the size of a finger joint called facets. There are two at each spinal level (one on each side), which translates to 14 facet joints in your neck, 24 in your thoracic spine, and 10 in your low back. These joints limit and control motion, so for example, this is one reason you can't turn your head around 360 degrees in *Exorcist* style (the cervical facets stop you at about 90 degrees of rotation).

One of the reasons to know about these joints is that they can be injured through trauma or get arthritis with wear and tear and cause pain and wreak havoc. For example, when they're painful, they

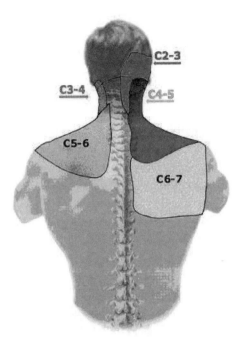

frequently shut down the local stabilizer muscles, causing instability and more wear and tear at that level. They're also good at referring pain to various areas. Look at the facet pain referral map, to the right, that shows where the various neck joints can project their pain. For example, if you have pain in a C2–C3 cervical facet (near the top of your neck), it will cause headaches. Or a C6–C7 facet joint near the bottom of your neck will cause shoulder blade pain. Finally, a lower back facet can also cause pain referred down the leg.

Because these joints are buried deep in the spine, unlike a painful finger joint, they can be difficult for the doctor to feel. As a result, finding out which one is hurting and in need of regenerative therapies to help the painful joint can oftentimes be difficult through an exam. As a result, the doctor may use a diagnostic block to help decide which joint hurts. As above, this is just numbing the suspected joint to make sure your pain goes away.

Radiofrequency: Nuking the Spine Joint Nerves to Take Away Pain

Radiofrequency ablation has become a common way to treat painful or injured neck and back facet joints. The nerve that takes pain signals from the joint is burned away using a needle with a tip that heats up. Based on the published research, this can be an effective way to help pain for more than a year in the neck and about 6-9 months in the low back. However, these nerves are there for a reason, so "nuking" the nerve should only be done when there's no other good option for treatment for the patient. We've had success in treating many patients with platelet or stem cell injections into these joints, which doesn't impact the facet joint nerves. In addition, in the low back, these nerves also supply the multifidus muscle, so burning the nerve can lead to atrophy of this stabilizing muscle and muscle-related instability in the spine.

Joints in the Upper Back: Where the Ribs Attach to the Spine

In many patients that fall or get hit in a car crash, we see pain at specific spots of their upper back or chest. Oftentimes the ribs as a cause get completely overlooked, other than a vague diagnosis of costochondritis (inflammation of the ribs) and a script for anti-inflammatories. Is there more to this problem?

The ribs attach to the spine at two joints each in the back and one in the front. These ribs move when you take a deep breath by expanding out like a bucket handle being lifted. They move from these pivot points in the back and the front. At these spots, strong ligaments connect the ribs to the spine and the breastbone (sternum). The most frequent type of injury we see is when the

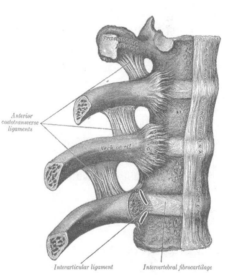

metal stiffeners in the back of car seats (meant to prevent the collapse of the seat back) hit these rib anchor spots in a rear-end car crash. This often loosens the ligaments that hold the ribs, causing spot pain in the back that gets worse with breathing or twisting. The front rib attachments can get injured by the air bag or the chest wall hitting something, causing similar pain areas. Another common cause of front rib pain is open heart surgery, where the rib joints get injured once the chest is "cracked." We usually treat these issues by tightening these ligaments with prolotherapy spiked with platelet growth factors.

Cutting Out Pieces: Helpful Debridement or a Slippery Slope to More Rapid Arthritis?

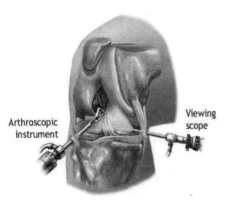

Arthroscopic instrument

Viewing scope

Often with only a cursory exam and a picture (which you now know may not show the cause of pain), our modern orthopedic care system schedules surgery. A common procedure used to help "clean up" a joint, like the knee, hip, shoulder, or ankle, is called <u>arthroscopic debridement</u>. The concept is that the surgeon will cut out loose pieces of cartilage, meniscus, or other tissues. While this may make some sense at face value, the tissues we're removing in debridement are made up of live cells often critical for the overall health of the joint. <u>Two large studies have shown that this surgery in the knee produces no better results than a fake placebo surgery or physical therapy</u>. Why? We're removing structure from the joint. Let's take an example. Say you owned a house where one day one of the walls started to crack and fall apart (like the meniscus seen on MRI), but the house is still structurally sound. You can repair the wall or remove the wall. Since you don't have the technology to repair the wall (which is what happens in many of today's joint surgeries— words like "repair" are actually a misnomer, and they often mean "cut out"), you decide to remove it. You may get some temporary benefit from removing the wall as it was an eyesore, and perhaps removing it makes the house flow better. However, since it's a load-bearing wall (helping to hold up the second story), things in the long run get worse. The floor on the second story starts to sag, and other walls begin to crack under loads they weren't designed to handle. Before long, it's clear that removing the wall was a bad idea. This is exactly what happens in many of today's modern joint surgeries. In the knee, we remove chunks of supporting meniscus with each surgery, <u>despite the fact that research has shown that doing so means that arthritis will likely develop much more quickly</u>.

How about surgery for a meniscus tear? Surely this must help as this is one of the most common surgeries performed in the United States today. Not so much. In fact, two recent studies question whether this procedure helps more than a placebo surgery. In one study, the surgery to remove a small part of the torn meniscus (often described by surgeons as surgery to "fix" the meniscus tear) was no better than physical therapy. In another recent study, the meniscus surgery was found to be no better than a fake surgery. You would think that we have a large body of scientific evidence that other common orthopedic surgeries are effective. We don't. In fact, we don't have high levels of scientific evidence that hip arthroscopy, rotator cuff repair, or low-back surgery is effective. Same with surgeries on the ankle, elbow, hand, and neck.

Is there a better way? Rather than cutting out tissue, our practice was the first in the United States to pioneer a new approach starting in 2005. We began using the patient's own stem cells in an attempt to heal damaged tissues rather than surgically removing the tissues. There's even a nice little video that helps to explain why we think this approach is better. Click on the image below to play that video.

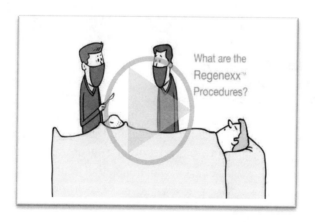

Understanding the Body's Repairmen: Stem Cells

Remember that house in your neighborhood that was inhabited by an older person who couldn't keep up with the maintenance? We'd all accept at face value that a house left unattended for years will weather and begin to slowly degrade and fall apart. Our joints and bodies are the same. A quick run around the block, a workout in the gym, or just daily use will cause microdamage in any number of tissues. Left unrepaired, these areas will begin to break down over time (just like the unattended house down the street).

So, what keeps us from falling apart after just a few years? The figure to the left tells the story of the opposing forces of damage versus repair. Everything we do every day adds small (or large) amounts of damage or wear and tear on our tissues. On the other side of that coin is repair. This is the mechanism that fixes the damage. When these two systems are equally matched (our repair system can easily keep up with the damage), you have healthy joints.

Turns out we have billions to trillions of tiny little repairmen in all the tissues of our body. These repairmen are called <u>adult stem cells</u>. As an example,

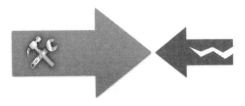

Young or Older and Healthy Joint: Repair abilities far exceed wear and tear.

consider an adult stem cell type called a <u>mesenchymal stem cell (MSC)</u>. These cells live in your tissues and are called into action once damage is detected. They can act as a general contractor in the repair response, giving signals to activate other subcontractor cell types

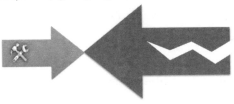

Older or Unhealthy Joint: Wear and tear exceeds repair abilities.

that are needed for the repair job or even firing (deactivating) cells that may be causing trouble. They can also "differentiate" (turn into) the final cell type needed for the repair. For example, if the cells are repairing the cartilage of your knee, they can differentiate into these cartilage cells. When we're young, while there may be a lot of abuse on the body, in general, the amount of repair capability (adult stem cell numbers and function) generally far exceeds the amount of damage we can inflict. <u>As we age, we have fewer of these stem cells around</u>. Even when we're younger, an area can become injured so that it doesn't allow the repairmen in the door (less blood flow, or there just aren't enough cells to affect a proper repair). At this point, the amount of damage starts to exceed the body's ability to repair.

What if we could turn that equation around? What if, despite being older or even younger with an area that has too much damage for the local repair cells to handle, we could amplify repair in the area? As you might have guessed, this is a basic tenant of Orthopedics 2.0. The doctor's job is to increase the local repair response in nonhealing tissues so that it exceeds the existing damage or wear and tear on the area. This also includes the other side of the coin—the doctor should avoid prescribing or injecting medication that will harm or slow this repair process. In addition, the final part of the doctor's job is to reduce the local damage on the area. How is this done?

Improving the Repair Response

We can divide increasing the repair response into approaches with three levels of sophistication.

- Level I: Microinjury
- Level 2: Improving the Healing Environment Level 3: Stem Cells

Level 1: Microinjury

Ever since ancient times, creating a small injury to prompt healing has been seen as a good idea. For horses, this was called "<u>pin firing</u>." The technique was to take a hot poker and place it into a nonhealing ligament to cause small amounts of damage to the area, which caused the body to kick up a repair response. While barbaric, it generally worked. For centuries doctors have created small injuries in a nonhealing wound by "roughing" up the tissues. Physicians still use this concept today for tendons, ligaments, and joint capsules. For example, in a <u>shoulder capsulorrhaphy</u>, a surgeon usually inserts a small catheter that heats the tissue to prompt healing in a damaged

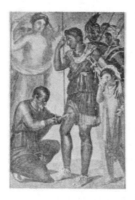

shoulder capsule (the covering of the shoulder joint that helps control motion). Doctors still score ligaments with scalpels and beat up tendons with a needle (percutaneous tenotomy), all to prompt a healing response. Another example is microfracture surgery, which is a procedure used to treat a hole in the cartilage in a damaged joint. In this surgery, the doctor pokes holes in the bone to cause the cartilage to heal. Finally, the procedure known as prolotherapy is in this same category. In this procedure, rather than a mechanical injury being initiated, the physician injects a chemical irritant to cause a chemical microinjury. All of these types of treatment rely on the same concept, that we get one bite of the healing "apple," and if something fails to heal completely the first time, we can create more bites at that apple simply by causing a small injury to the area.

The big advantage to microinjury techniques is that these basic procedures are simple and often inexpensive. The downside is that while many times they work well, sometimes they don't have enough "oomph" to produce the right type of healing or enough healing. In addition, they also tend to do better when fibrous tissue repair is what's needed. This means they can heal ligaments and tendons with much the same composition as the original tissue, but for things like cartilage, they produce inferior-quality tissue. For example, for microfracture, it's been well known for years that lower quality fibrocartilage is predominantly produced rather than true hyaline cartilage.

The Original Level I Regenerative Injection Technique: Prolotherapy

Prolotherapy is an injection method where chemicals are injected to cause a small inflammatory healing reaction. In the 1940s, this was a mainstream orthopedic procedure used to treat lax ligaments and spinal pain. Heck, it even had its own pharmaceutical (Sanusol). However, in the next half of the twentieth century, prolotherapy fell out of favor. Why? Some say it was linked to the bad outcome of a single injection placed where it shouldn't be in the spinal canal. However, others place prolotherapy's demise on the fact that it had no sustainable medical business model. It was simply replaced by big surgical procedures that were far sexier and had better reimbursement through a new concept at the time—employer-sponsored medical insurance. While we may never know what happened, over the past two decades, I've seen this simple and inexpensive technique work for patients who otherwise would not have been helped. I've published on prolotherapy's ability to tighten loose spine ligaments simply through injection, and others have published on the same observation in lax knee ligaments.

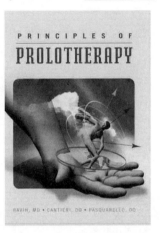

If you have a loose ligament, prolotherapy may be a good option. However, like any regenerative injection technique, accuracy of placement matters. As a result, prolotherapy should almost always be performed under imaging guidance, especially when deep specific structures are being treated. I wrote an article on this topic a few years back that explains how this works.

Level II: Improving the Healing Environment

The next level of sophistication beyond just creating a healing microinjury is making the conditions in the area more conducive to healing, or *anabolic*. You may have heard this term associated with body builders who use steroids. This is not the same use here, although body builders "build" muscle, so this is why they use anabolic steroid (literally, "steroids that build"). Here the term means making an area pro-repair, or better able to heal.

Creating an anabolic healing environment is not a new concept in medicine and surgery. For centuries, physicians have known that some people have better innate abilities to heal, while others have fewer healing capabilities. The acronym PPP (piss-poor protoplasm) was used in my medical school training to mean a patient who, due to disease or extreme old age, was unable to heal after surgery. While surgeons have always known that some patients could have a compromised ability to heal, not much attention has been paid in how to make routine and otherwise healthy patients heal better. Doctors have always understood the basics, like good nutrition, young age, high levels of fitness, and good blood supply. About 20 years ago, that started to change in the dental community. Some dentists began experimenting with a simple concoction called PRP (platelet-rich plasma). The dentists used this stuff made from their patients' own blood to help dental implants heal.

PRP is a simple example of how we can improve the healing environment. Your blood has platelets that contain growth factors that help to ramp up healing. To understand how these platelets work, a paper cut will illustrate the basic points. When we cut ourselves, we bleed into the cut. The blood coagulates because of cell fragments that live in our blood called platelets. The job of the platelets doesn't stop there. They go on to release certain growth factors that stimulate local cells to heal the cut.

Growth factors are like espresso shots for cells. A cell works at a certain pace to do its job. If we add growth factors (like those in PRP), it's like buying all of the cells trying to repair the area a bunch of Starbucks gift cards. The cells react to the growth factors like people react to triple espresso shots: they work harder and faster. So, if we use an example of a construction site where we have a few bricklayers building a new wall, and we add growth factors (espresso shots), our bricklayers will build our wall faster.

As you might have guessed, Orthopedics 2.0 uses these same concepts to promote healing. The most basic level II procedure today is PRP, which can be mixed up from a patient blood sample in a bedside centrifuge or in a simple hospital or clinic-based lab. PRP means that the healing platelets have been concentrated. Injecting the patient's own blood can often accomplish the same thing, as it's also rich in platelets.

Regenexx Uses a Flexible Lab Platform

In this section, you'll see some amazing things we can create and use to help healing. Most physicians use small bedside machines to create some of these things, and others can't be created outside of a lab. The advantage of these small bedside machines is that they are easy to use as all you need to know is where to place the sample and where the "On" button is located. The disadvantage is that they are "one size fits all" devices that only create one thing. Hence, we have long since gone to what we call a *flexible lab platform*. This means that we use validated protocols in an in-office lab. This is more expansive and more difficult for the doctor, but the advantage to the patient is fantastic. Meaning, we can create more things with more customization for the patient. For more information, click on the video below:
https://youtu.be/jAVu8Erk-qA

Not All PRP Is Created Equal

One of our focus areas since 2005 has been figuring out how to use various forms of PRP to get stem cells to grow better. This extensive experience has led us to understand that there are different "flavors" of PRP and that some of them seem to work better for kicking stem cells into high gear. How can you tell the difference? Look at the color of the PRP. Based on our lab data, red PRP doesn't work as well as amber PRP to promote stem cell activity. Most automatic bedside centrifuges used by doctors today produce this red, bloody PRP.

Why is red PRP a problem? It's rich in red and white blood cells. When it comes to energizing stem cells toward repairing more tissue, our lab experiments show that red PRP doesn't have the same "espresso shot" kick as PRP without red and white cells (amber PRP). Based on these experiments, we have created what we call a "super concentrated platelet" procedure (SCP) to maximally stimulate stem cells into action. Click here for an infographic that explains the issues and lab data in more detail. In addition, click on the video link below to see a two-minute animation that explains these differences.

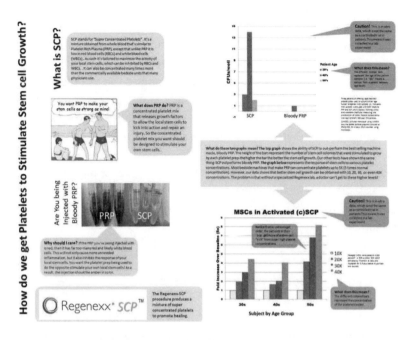

The other big difference with SCP is that since we create it by hand in our Flexible Lab Platform for every patient in a lab rather than mass manufacturing it in an automated push-button centrifuge, we have much more control over the composition of the final preparation. In particular, while most bedside centrifuges can only concentrate to about 5-7 times

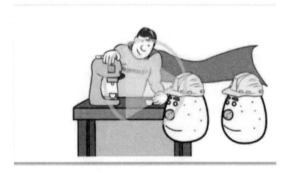

more platelets than are normally present in the blood, we can concentrate SCP all the way up to 40 times over baseline! Is getting to higher platelet concentrations better? Yes, with this type of PRP, we see more activity in local stem cells with higher concentrations of platelets. <u>For this lab data, click here</u>.

In our clinic, we also use next-generation level II tools beyond PRP. These include platelet lysate (PL). In the case of PL, our advanced cell biology lab makes PRP from the patient's blood and then breaks open the platelets to make all of the growth factors immediately available.

The difference between PRP (or SCP as we call it) and PL is the same as between a time- release pill and an immediate-release pill. PRP has whole platelets that release their growth factors over time. PL has all of the growth factors immediately available. Based on our experience, there are specific reasons to use one or the other. For example, in our clinical experience, PL is excellent to use around nerves.

We can also produce newer types of platelet lysate (fourth generation). In our lab experiments, we noticed that despite blowing up platelet bodies and releasing growth factors, there were still some whole platelets left. This meant that there were still growth factors to be released. As a result, we developed a proprietary type of triple lysate that gets all of the available growth factors out of the platelets.

Can We Create a PRP That's Better at Making Cartilage?

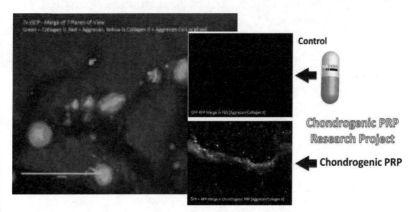

Control

Chondrogenic PRP
Research Project

Chondrogenic PRP

Since PRP is often used in joints, and one of the major regenerative medicine concerns there is healing cartilage, is PRP good at cartilage repair? One of the growth factors in PRP is TGF-beta, which is very good at helping cartilage grow. However, PRP also contains a soup of growth factors, some of which may or may not promote cartilage repair. As a result, we have been researching this issue for some time and have created novel platelet mixes that are better at helping stem cells make cartilage in lab experiments (see illustration above that shows that our chondrogenic PRP produces more cartilage components than a control in the lab—the green is cartilage being made).

How about SCP? We have tested our SCP in the lab for its ability to promote stem cells to produce cartilage and found it to be very capable of this feat (see fluorescent microscopy image above).

Regenokine or Orthokine

In Europe, there has been a blood-based treatment called "Orthokine" for many years. In the U.S., this has been rebranded as "Regenokine." It involves taking blood from the patient and then prompting the white blood cells to produce a natural anti-inflammatory chemical called interleukin receptor protein antagonist (IRAP). The idea is that this natural substance will reduce arthritis symptoms. In fact, you may have heard Kobe Bryant went to Europe to get this injected.

How good is Orthokine? Studies done by the company have shown that it barely beats a placebo for treating knee arthritis symptoms. In fact, a PRP injection would be better based on comparing the data. While we don't use this product, our flexible lab platform can mix up a natural anti-inflammatory cocktail that may help some patients who have more inflammation associated with their arthritis.

A2M: Alpha-2-Macroglobulin

One of the more interesting developments of the past several years has been the discovery of an anti-breakdown molecule called alpha-2-macroglobulin (A2M). In animals, this seems to block or use up the inflammatory chemicals in a joint that can lead to arthritic joint destruction. While this has never been documented to slow the progression of arthritis in humans, this type of therapy may show promise.

Given our flexible lab platform can create an A2M-enriched serum from the patient's blood, we have begun using this cytokine. Where we see it perform well is in patients who have more inflammation with their arthritis. We have also begun to offer it to patients who want to try to stave off the progression of joint destruction. Will this work? Only time will tell.

Level III: Stem Cell Therapy or Adding in the General Contractors of the Body

While level I therapy is about causing a little injury to prompt healing and level II about getting the local cells to work harder or controlling inflammation, level III is about adding more workers to the area. Staying with our construction-site metaphor, a general contractor (GC) is the person who pulls a construction project together. He or she hires subcontractors, like plumbers, carpenters, and electricians. Does your body have a GC cell that can help coordinate its daily repair jobs?

The GC's of your body are stem cells. So, level III advanced techniques use concentrated or cultured stem cells to help repair tissues. There are a number of different types of stem cells. We've all heard of embryonic stem cells

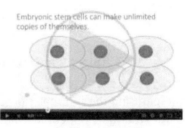

Embryonic stem cells can make unlimited copies of themselves.

that are taken from a growing embryo. While these cells are very potent stem cells, they also have the nasty habit of forming tumors. To better understand why that happens, I've created a short video to the right (click to watch).

Cells can also be taken from umbilical cord or adult stem cells. However, while some of these cell types might be appropriate as last-ditch efforts to save someone's life, their risk of transmitting genetic disease makes them too risky for orthopedic applications. As an example, in one study, an older rat bred to have osteoporosis donated stem cells to a young rat without the disease. **The young rat acquired osteoporosis in the bargain!** Since we currently don't

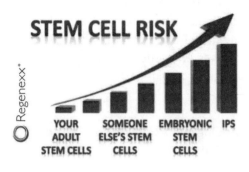

possess the technology to screen donors for all inheritable diseases, the risk of using someone else's stem cells is too high for now (in my opinion). Please also note that, as discussed earlier, commercially available amniotic or umbilical cord products that providers tell you have millions of live and viable stem cells are dead tissue products. More on this in a bit.

Finally, the newest stem cell types are called induced pluripotent stem cells (iPS or iPSCs) or stimulus-triggered acquired pluripotency (STAP). While all of this sounds very daunting, the basic concept is that these are artificial stem cells that don't exist in nature, created from natural cells. These are created by heavy-handed genetic manipulation of the normal cells from STAP, click here to watch the video.

Fat vs. Bone Marrow Stem Cells

Anyone perusing the Internet can see that there are two stem cell types from the same patient (aka autologous) that seem ubiquitous: fat and bone marrow stem cells. When we began using stem cells in 2005, we investigated which of these we should use. At the time, there was mounting evidence that bone marrow stem cells had real utility in orthopedic applications and very little data published showing that fat stem cells were very helpful.

Before delving into that research, let's review the five most common procedures being offered in autologous stem cells for orthopedic injuries (illustration on next page).

As you can see on the next page, there are two different bone marrow procedures (same-day and advanced) and three different fat procedures (two same-day and one advanced). The same-day bone

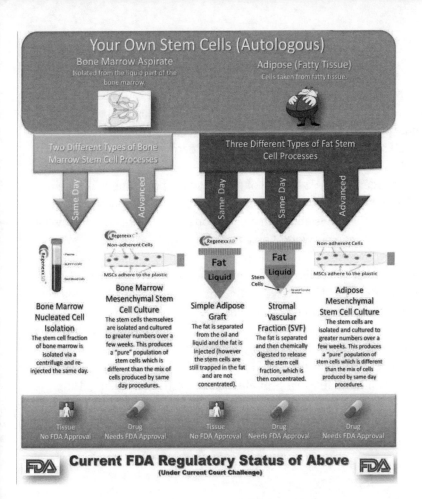

marrow procedure is equivalent to the Regenexx-SD procedure, and the advanced bone marrow procedure is Regenexx-C[1] where cells are cultured for two weeks. On the fat stem cell side, there's a simple adipose fat graft. We have developed our version of this procedure that includes microfragmented fat, which maximizes the number of stem cells, but so that the procedure remains compliant with FDA regulations. In addition, there's another fat-based procedure where the cells are digested away from the tissue that holds them in place.

---

[1] The Regenexx-C cultured stem cell procedure is only offered through independently owned and operated medical services providers operating exclusively outside the United States. These service providers are not part of or affiliated with the Centeno-Schultz Clinic or any US Regenexx Network provider. The Regenexx-C procedure is not approved by the FDA for use in the United States.

This is called *stromal vascular fraction* (SVF), and, regrettably, this is not currently legal for clinical use in the U.S. In fact, the FDA has cracked down on several clinics using this procedure with intravenous injections to try to cure a multitude of diseases. Finally, just like in the bone marrow procedures, you can culture the cells to get more, so there is an adipose advanced procedure. So now that you know what's being offered, can research guide us as to which is better researched for orthopedic use—bone marrow or fat? Every year I search the US Library of Medicine for publications on the use of different cell types to treat orthopedic conditions. This year's version still shows about an eight to one edge for research showing that bone marrow works versus fat.

How about a comparison of how the cells are harvested? Bone marrow stem cells are taken from the patient using a bone marrow aspiration. This is where a small hole is poked through the bone with a special needle. Fat stem cells are harvested during liposuction where fat is collected through a cannula. As you can see from the graph to the right, the risk of liposuction is about 21 times more than that of a bone marrow aspirate. Again, on the safety of getting the

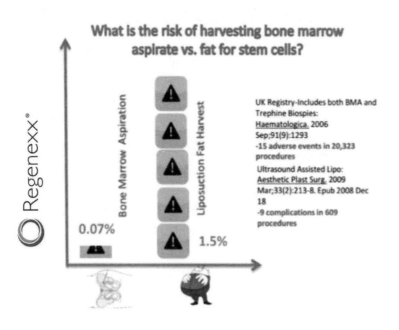

What is the risk of harvesting bone marrow aspirate vs. fat for stem cells?

Bone Marrow Aspiration — 0.07%

Liposuction Fat Harvest — 1.5%

UK Registry-Includes both BMA and Trephine Biospies: Haematologica, 2006 Sep;91(9):1293
-15 adverse events in 20,323 procedures

Ultrasound Assisted Lipo: Aesthetic Plast Surg, 2009 Mar;33(2):213-8. Epub 2008 Dec 18
-9 complications in 609 procedures

Regenexx®

cells from the patient, bone marrow stem cells win again.

In summary, there is still much more data supporting the use of bone marrow to treat orthopedic diseases. Might that change with time? It may, but for now, we'll go with what the data says is likely to be better for our patients.

Mesenchymal Stem Cells

There are many types of adult autologous stem cells, but for the purposes of this orthopedics discussion, one stands out as the best candidate for our general contractor position: the mesenchymal stem cell (MSC). These cells are found in many tissues (for example, as above, they are found in bone marrow aspirate and fat). For orthopedic applications, their ability to help coordinate the repair response as well as turn into cartilage, bone, tendon, muscle, and ligament make them ideal. Other cells, such as very small embryonic-like or embryonic-like stem cells (VSELs or ELSCs), are also promising for orthopedic use, but not enough research has been done yet on these adult stem cell types with regard to safety to make them practical for everyday use. In addition, some prominent researchers don't even believe that they exist. Also realize that there are likely hundreds of classes and subclasses of adult stem cells that will eventually be used for therapy. Many of these may even be combined with mixtures of other non-stem cells or tissue-engineered scaffolds to better promote healing.

Does Where and How You Get Your Bone Marrow Matter?

First, when most patients hear about a bone marrow procedure, they think of a different procedure than the one we perform (a bone marrow biopsy is the one you've heard about, while we perform a bone marrow aspiration [BMA]). A BMA is a simple procedure where the area is thoroughly numbed, and then a needle is gently worked through the bone to pull out what looks like thick blood. Is this really painful? In 2007, we polled our patients and found out that about 9 in 10 thought it was no big deal.

Second, where you take the marrow can make a big difference in the number of cells you get. For example, recently some doctors who aren't comfortable using more advanced guidance techniques have begun taking it from below the knee rather than from the back of the hip. Regrettably, <u>this knee site doesn't produce as many cells as the hip site</u>; hence, we use the hip procedure that yields more stem cells.

Third, how you take bone marrow is **critical**. For example, many doctors shortcut this procedure because it's easier for them, but this robs the sample of stem cell content. The problem? Taking small amounts of bone marrow aspirate from many sites will yield many more stem cells. Taking more marrow from a single site reduces stem cells and causes more peripheral blood contamination (which doesn't contain stem cells). This is because the bone marrow space communicates freely with the vascular system. How many doctors perform a bone marrow aspiration procedure correctly? In my experience, 5–10% of those performing this procedure use the more time-intensive approach.

ECM: Extracellular Matrix

Sometimes, when we think the tissue we are injecting into is more beat-up or torn or has a gap, we will inject an extracellular matrix (ECM). This is a noncellular tissue that can both prompt healing itself and act as a scaffold for cells. A good example of this is using amniotic membrane. While certain clinics trying to scam patients will claim that this tissue has live stem cells, it's actually nonviable. Hence, we use it with real stem cells (or PRP) to help promote healing in specific clinical scenarios.

Other ECM products we may use include DBM (demineralized bone) or animal-derived basement membrane. The first tissue type is bone that has had the cells removed and has been turned into a gel, paste, or powder. It's osteoinductive (meaning it gives cells the chemical clue to become bone) and acts as a place where cells can grow. We will generally use this when there is a gap in bone like a nonhealing fracture. The second product is one that has been shown to be helpful in muscle repair.

Different Orthopedic Stem Cell Procedures

As discussed above, there are two different bone marrow stem cell procedures—one is same day and the other is cultured. What's the difference? The same-day procedure is what it sounds like. The stem cells are isolated and used the same day. The cultured procedure grows the stem cells to bigger numbers over a few weeks.

Almost all same-day procedures being used today are with bone marrow processed in automatic bedside machines that remove one fraction of the bone marrow that is rich in stem cells—the buffy coat. The issue with these machines is that they often can't be very exact, so they also isolate a lot of junk cells with the stem cells. As a result, we only perform this process of extracting the stem cells by hand using our flexible lab platform so it can be accomplished with more precision.

The buffy coat has both the MSCs, discussed above, as well as hematopoietic stem cells (HSCs). While the MSCs are good for helping to repair orthopedic tissues, in our clinical experience, the HSCs are good at bringing in new blood supply. This can be very important for tissues like the meniscus or rotator cuff where poor blood supply may be a cause for delayed healing. Other research has shown that they may serve a key role in muscle repair. Both of these cell types make up the Regenexx-SD procedure, which is often used to treat less-severe arthritis; meniscus tears; labral tears; and tendon/muscle tears, like rotator cuff.

Our dedication to lab research has also allowed us to advance this same- day procedure way beyond where it has been. We discovered a second fraction in the bone marrow that's very rich in stem cells and is currently being discarded by everyone else. This layer has many more stem cells per unit volume than the buffy coat, and our lab research shows that they're fast growing and very useful for orthopedic purposes. As a result, we've increased the number of stem cells we can pull out of the bone marrow by a factor of five to seven by isolating this new fraction. When we compare how many stem cells we're able to isolate in the lab per unit volume to the number that automatic bedside machines can isolate, it's 15–20 times more!

How effective are these same-day stem cell procedures? I can answer that question with the large amount of data we have collected and continue to amass every month. Please follow with me online with our registry-based outcome tool. What's this?

Throughout our website, you'll see references to live outcome data. Depending on where you're coming from, you may or may not get to choose which joint (above). However, by using this web-based app, you can see how patients in aggregate do with our procedures.

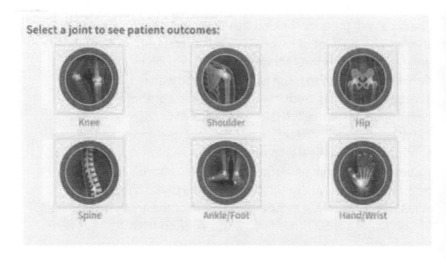

Regenexx Live Patient Outcome Data

In general, you'll see nice decreases in pain and increases in function, like this graph for almost 8,500 patients with knee arthritis:

Does this mean that the procedure helped everyone? Absolutely not! It does show, in my opinion, that this approach of using same-day stem cells to treat knee arthritis is viable. For more information on this data, click here for live patient outcome data.

Why do we have this data when everyone else seems to have very little? We have been investing in data collection through a treatment registry since 2005 and now have the most patients tracked through a registry and treated with stem cells in the world. Also realize that this data only applies to the Regenexx procedure and not to other stem cell procedures that use other cell types or other isolation methods from bone marrow or fat. For example, for knee arthritis, our proprietary SD procedure protocol uses a preinjection (to use a farming metaphor, this is "till the soil"), a stem cell reinject (plant the seeds), and a postinjection (fertilize).

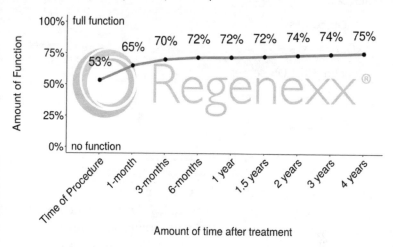

Amount of time after treatment

In addition, our biostatistics staff has been able to start to slice and dice the data to glean information that may be helpful in guiding treatment decisions. For example, our knee data shows that <u>your arthritis severity</u> (meaning if your arthritis is mild or severe) doesn't predict how well or poorly you will do with a same-day Regenexx-SD stem cell treatment. In addition, <u>your age doesn't seem to matter either</u> (i.e., older patients do as well as younger patients). In addition, <u>being heavier doesn't seem to hurt outcome</u>. All of this is important because for many surgical procedures used to treat arthritis, the severity, your age, and
your weight do matter.

We haven't only been collecting data from our patients with knee arthritis. We've also been tracking patients with arthritis in many joints as well as with more specific problems. For example, patients with hip arthritis with good versus poor range of motion and patients who have tears in their knee ACL or shoulder rotator cuff, who receive precise injections into these tears either under fluoroscopy or ultrasound guidance. In addition, we track patients who have arthritis in their thumbs or arthritis in the main joint of the ankle (tibiotalar). How do other joints and problems fare with same-day stem cells? Find out by reviewing our <u>live outcome tool</u> by body area at the following links:

- <u>Shoulder Outcomes</u>
- <u>Back/Spine Outcomes</u>
- <u>Knee Outcomes</u>
- <u>Hip Outcomes</u>
- <u>Hand and Wrist Outcomes</u>
- <u>Foot and Ankle Outcomes</u>
- <u>Elbow Outcomes</u>

Randomized Controlled Trials

The gold standard of research is what's called a randomized controlled trial (RCT). This is a clinical study of a treatment where patients are randomly assigned to be in one group versus the other. In our case, we have a group that gets the stem treatment and one that gets standard physical therapy. Then at some point, if the patients in the therapy group aren't improving, they can cross over to the stem cell treatment group.

We have three RCTs with results at this point. They are in knee arthritis, knee ACL tears, and shoulder rotator cuff tears. All three show excellent results versus the physical therapy group. The outcomes from the knee arthritis trial are shown here. This data has been submitted for peer-reviewed publication. Again, why doesn't anyone else have this data? They haven't spent the time and resources to test what they do.

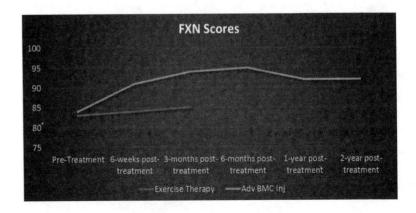

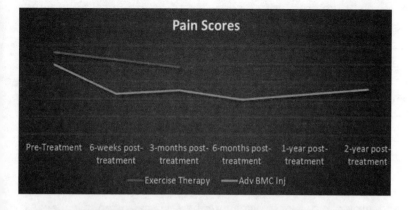

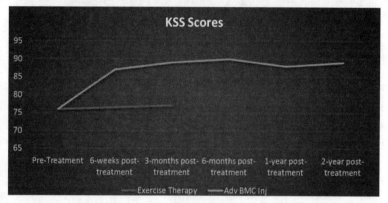

Can We Do More with a Same-Day Stem Cell Procedure?

In 2006, our clinic pioneered a new approach to stem cells, culturing them to grow more. In this advanced procedure, we can obtain about 20–50 times more stem cells than in our same-day procedure. This Regenexx-C[2] method has been the subject of <u>several safety papers published in the U.S. National Library of Medicine</u>. The cultured stem cell injections were much safer than the more invasive surgical procedures they helped patients avoid. The outcome data also shows that the higher number of cultured stem cells tend to work a bit better than same-day stem cells.

---

[2] The Regenexx-C cultured stem cell procedure is only offered through independently owned and operated medical services providers operating exclusively outside the United States. These service providers are not part of or affiliated with the Centeno-Schultz Clinic or any US Regenexx Network provider. The Regenexx-C procedure is not approved by the FDA for use in the United States.

Where might we use cultured versus same-day stem cells? In our experience, for certain applications, cultured stem cells are helpful, while for others, there is only a small difference. For example, in patients with more severe thumb and hip arthritis, cultured cells seem to be significantly better than same-day stem cells. However, for many applications, like tendon/ligament and bone healing, there seems to be a smaller difference. In addition, for knee arthritis, there may only be a small advantage to using cultured cells.

One big advantage to cultured cells is the ability to save them for future use in cryopreservation (deep freeze). In addition, since these cells are grown in culture to bigger numbers, we can often save many treatments for the same joint or other future injuries.

Is Either Stem Cell Procedure Growing a Bunch of New Cartilage?

We've taken many before and after research-grade MRIs of knees and other joints where stem cells have been successfully used to treat more severe arthritis. While some show some major changes, most don't. So what's happening? We hypothesize that a bad joint with arthritis is catabolic (meaning it has a toxic stew of chemicals that break down cartilage). It gets this way because many of the stem cells that live in the joint to maintain a healthy environment are gone. When we perform a cultured stem cell injection, we're replacing this "stem cell reserve" (stem cells whose job it is to keep the joint healthy). This then turns the chemical environment in the joint anabolic (healthy). Click here to learn more about this topic.

Stem cells also work in many other ways outside of turning into new cartilage. Take, for example, the concept of exosomes. These tiny little packets are excreted by stem cells and can contains snippets of mRNA (an instruction sheet to make proteins). A stem cell can use these mRNA protein instruction sheets to task another cell to make proteins on its behalf. For a short one-minute video explanation on the topic, click here.

Stem cells can additionally work through what's called paracrine effects. This means that the stem cell excretes chemical messages called cytokines. Think of the stem cell as a general contractor who is involved in coordinating a repair of tissue. It barks out orders to hire subcontractor cells to do some of the work. While cells can't talk, their version is releasing very specific chemicals that can attract the types of cells it needs and then releasing other chemicals to give basic instructions to the other cells. For a short video that explains this, click on the video link above.

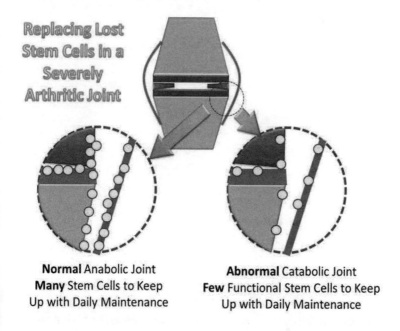

Replacing Lost Stem Cells in a Severely Arthritic Joint

Normal Anabolic Joint
Many Stem Cells to Keep
Up with Daily Maintenance

Abnormal Catabolic Joint
Few Functional Stem Cells to Keep
Up with Daily Maintenance

More recently, <u>one interesting study also explained another mechanism for how stem cells may help arthritic joints</u>. In the type of catabolic joints that I describe above, there are cells that act like Pac-Man by gobbling up normal, healthy cartilage (aka activated macrophages). These cells are deactivated by mesenchymal stem cells and, as such, stop eating the good cartilage.

I've also done a short one-minute video on how this Pac-Man cell inhibition works. For that, <u>click here</u>.

Wait, I Went to a Seminar Where They Showed Us Before and After X-Rays Showing That Lots of New Cartilage Had Been Regrown!

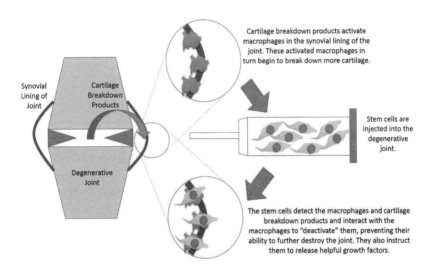

As discussed above, this is a scam. <u>Regrettably, if you tilt the X-ray beam even a few degrees, this will make it appear that you have more or less cartilage.</u> All of these X-rays that we have examined have obvious evidence of tilting of the X-ray beam. Take a look at my knee below where we tilted the beam. In one image I appear to have less cartilage, and in another it appears that I have more (taken just seconds apart).

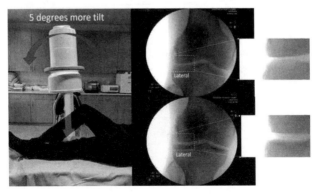

Bone: The Structure of the Joint

Bone is the structure that gives form to the joint—a place where two bones meet. Ligaments and muscles help keep the bones aligned, and cartilage acts as their cushion. When the joint suffers from arthritis, the cartilage breaks down, reducing the cushion. But can the bone develop issues too?

While we think of bone as cement, it's actually like hard plastic that gives and absorbs shock. However, it relies on the cartilage to help it work properly as a machine to mitigate forces. When that cartilage is damaged, the bone can swell.

Bone swelling is called a bone marrow lesion (BML) and is readily seen on certain types of MRI images as a bright spot. These areas are places where microfractures have occurred. In addition, research shows that while these areas of bone swelling may be caused by poor cartilage not absorbing the forces of the joint, the swelling of the bone may also cause more cartilage damage. Can this problem be helped? We have seen good results with what we call percutaneous stem-cell-assisted subchondroplasty (PSCAS). This involves careful mapping of the lesion using MRI and then placing a needle into the bone and injecting stem cells to shore up the area. By helping the bone, in this technique, we believe we can help the cartilage.
Note, again, that this procedure (shown below in a knee cap bone) is much more sophisticated than what you will see in most clinics. Ninety-nine percent of the time, all that's done is a simple injection inside the knee joint (either blind or with ultrasound). Note that here there is an X-ray–guided injection into the specific area of the bone with the BML.

Bone and Joint Tissues Are Alive!

Why do bone spurs develop? Are they good or bad? We've come to think of bone as inanimate cement. However, bone is made up of mature cells (osteoblasts) and stem cells that react to their environment. It's well known, for instance, that when the cushioning cartilage in a joint wears out, the bone underneath the worn out cartilage makes itself thicker to handle the new forces. We know that people who don't exercise or who pursue non-weight-bearing exercise have more brittle bones, and that <u>people who lift heavy weights have more dense bones</u>. So bone is alive and quickly reacts to its environment. How quickly? As an example, for many years most physicians were convinced that bone spurs in the spine took years to form. This was based on the theory that bone was dumb, inanimate cement. <u>However, more-recent research shows that when the lumbar discs are injured as part of an experiment, bone spurs begin to form in the 1 to 2-month time frame.</u>

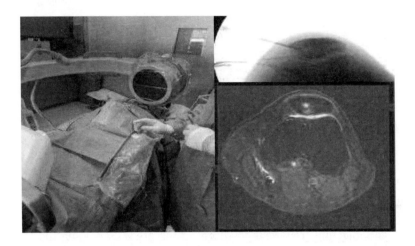

The same holds true for muscles, <u>tendons</u>, and <u>ligaments</u>. They all react to increased strain forces by making themselves thicker and stronger. This ability to react quickly to increased (or decreased) demands is mediated in part by adult stem cells. The switch from seeing these orthopedic tissues as inanimate filler (bone, cartilage) or pieces of inanimate duct tape (ligament, tendon) to living tissues that react is a key concept in understanding why alignment of the joints is so important in Orthopedics 2.0.

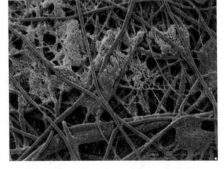

Functional Bone Spurs?

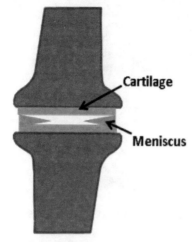

Cartilage

Meniscus

Knee Joint

Bone reacts to forces. I've spoken to many patients over the past few years who are planning to have surgery to remove <u>bone spurs</u>. I can think of a few situations where this makes a lot of sense, like when a bone spur is pressing on a nerve or severely limiting range of motion or rubbing on an important structure. I call these *nonfunctional bone spurs*.

However, in many situations, bone spurs are functional. What does this mean? Let's take the example of bone spurs that develop in a knee. The knee has <u>cartilage</u> and a <u>fibrocartilage meniscus</u> (spacer). Both the cartilage and meniscus components are shock absorbers with the meniscus also acting as pacer to help keep the joint surfaces apart. When the meniscus is healthy, it stays within the joint (see picture at top left). When the meniscus gets degenerated or pieces of the meniscus are removed surgically, the meniscus starts to migrate out of the joint (see picture top right next page). Since bone is alive and reacts to these forces, the body responds by placing bone in this area to take advantage of this new meniscus position (see picture to the bottom right). This response is called a "bone spur," or "osteophyte." We've been conditioned to believe that all bone spurs are bad. However, as you can see here, these bone spurs allow the knee to take advantage of this new meniscus position and continue to use the spacer (meniscus) to absorb shock. If we remove these bone spurs, the knee

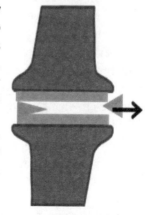

loses its ability to absorb shock, and the body will just place more bone spurs in this location. I call these "functional bone spurs" in that they serve a purpose and their removal doesn't positively impact the joint. Since all bone spurs are a reaction to instability or joint forces, we have to be careful about removing this reactive tissue to make sure that the joint will be better off after removal.

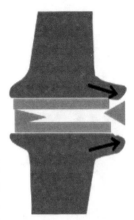

The Regenexx Difference

When we first pioneered orthopedic stem cell therapy in 2005, we were the only physicians in the United States doing this type of work. This last few years has seen a bevy of clinics opening and offering stem cell therapies for pretty much whatever ails you—from arthritis to ALS to COPD to MS. A few of these clinics are legitimately trying to do a good job, but most are not. How can you tell the difference? First, let's look at the clinic types that are popping up.

1.	The Miracle Fat Stem Cell Clinic: These types of clinics using SVF fat as their source of stem cells offer treatments for a multitude of diseases, which include knee and hip arthritis. They perform a small liposuction to get cells, and as such are usually run by a plastic surgeon who oversees a processing facility that distributes cells to other medical specialists. Some claim to be operating research studies, but when I have investigated these further, most of this is more sales than reality (e.g., one clinic system claimed to have an Institutional Review Board [IRB] research approval that turned out to have been rescinded). In addition, on the orthopedics side of the treatments, these are usually blind, nonspecific injections (without any guidance to ensure placement) somewhere in the vicinity of the painful joint. They frequently will combine these local injections with an IV infusion of fat stem cells, 97% of which will end up in the lungs and never see the joint. As you know from the previous discussion, fat stem cells don't work as well as marrow cells for orthopedic purposes, so the orthopedic side of the business seems to be an afterthought to drive revenue.

2.   The Little Bedside Machine Clinic: These clinics are often more focused on orthopedic problems, but use an automated bedside "one size fits all" machine to process bone marrow cells and platelet-rich plasma. Some of these clinics do offer guidance of the injection, but very little effort is placed on tracking patients or reporting outcome data. So, the type of treatment registry data that you've read about here isn't going to be reported by these clinics, leaving the patient to fly blind on how well these procedures work or don't work. These machines also produce about one-tenth to one-fifteenth of the stem cells per unit volume as a Regenexx-SD procedure (based on our lab studies). They also only isolate one fraction in the bone marrow that contains stem cells and discard the other fraction (not knowing that it has valuable cells).

3.   The Amniotic, Placental, or Umbilical Cord "Stem Cell" Clinic: These are usually chiropractic offices (but sometimes acupuncture or age-management outfits) that heavily advertise and hold many seminars. They usually hire a nurse to inject, as in most states, chiropractors and acupuncturists can't perform procedures. They also use commercially available amniotic, placental, or umbilical cord products and claim that these have millions of stem cells. However, all of these are regulated by the FDA to be dead tissue. In addition, our own research and that performed by a third-party nonprofit also confirmed that these products were nonviable and dead on arrival. Hence, claiming that these have millions of live and young stem cells makes this a scam. Why then do some patients report relief? These products contain growth factors like the platelets in your own blood. Hence, these can help reduce pain and prompt some repair, but we can get those same results using platelet-rich plasma made from your blood for a fraction of the price.

4.   The Orthopedic Surgery Fat or Amnio "Stem Cell" Clinic: This is usually a reputable orthopedic surgeon who doesn't know what he or she doesn't know. Surgeons learn much of what they know about new products from orthopedic sales reps. As with any sales cycle, what the salesmen tells the buyer and reality are often two different things. Hence, these surgeons have been sold the idea that the fat kit (usually Lipogems) that they use isolates stem cells. Regrettably, our research and that done by others doesn't show this to be the case (the stem cells are still locked in the fat). The same happens with

amniotic, placental, and umbilical cord tissue the surgeons are sold, the rep claims stem cells to make the sale, but this is not reality. Hence, all of these "little white sales lies" get passed on to the consumer. There is nothing malicious about these deceptions as the surgeon got zero training on any of this in medical school or residency, so everything he or she knows comes from a salesperson trying to move product.

5.   The "We Don't Need to Concentrate Marrow" Clinic: Since the '90s when the first bone marrow stem cells were used to treat bone disease in France, multiple studies have shown that concentrating the stem cells in marrow is linked to clinical outcome. This means that the more stem cells in the bone marrow, the better the patient fares with the treatment. However, recently a device manufacturer (Marrow Cellutions, also known through reseller names as Maxx-Regen) has begun suggesting this isn't needed. This is because they believe that their tool is so good at taking bone marrow that the bone marrow aspirate doesn't need to be concentrated in a machine. Since this is an attractive idea of saving time and resources, we tested these devices. Regrettably, we didn't find that the device worked as advertised, and, in fact, we found that concentrated marrow had far more stem cells than the stuff that came out of this magic doohickey. Hence, if a clinic uses these things, while you may do fine, if you have fewer stem cells due to age, you may be paying a lot of money for a substandard therapy.

So, what are the key components of a reputable clinic? I've provided a list below. All of this should be found on the website or by making a simple phone call. If you can't find it all, then run! More can be found on what to look for on clinic websites at this link.

A.	Treatment-registry tracking of patients
B.	Guidance of the injection
C.	A focus on orthopedic problems
D.	Candidacy grading
E.	Published research
F.	A customized approach to the processing of your tissue

G.   A clinical training and certification program for affiliates

Treatment Registry Tracking of Patients

Any new therapy that is standard of care needs to have data collected, even if it looks very promising from the standpoint of patient experience (e.g., a doctor says it has worked well in other patients). This means that standardized questionnaires are sent to the patient at set time points to see if they have less pain, more function, or had any complications with the procedure. This is a huge commitment on the part of the clinic and the doctor. As an example, right now we have a clinical research organization (CRO) quality, customized software to assist us in collecting data on the patients we have treated. We have a few full-time employees to collect data, several part-time supervisors, and a full-time biostatistician to analyze this data. When we want to report the data, we must enlist the help of expensive physicians to call patients who haven't responded to their questionnaires as this helps to make sure we have enough data to report. While we have a full-time biostatistician, we must also use more expensive doctor time to help our biostatistician decide what's clinically meaningful to analyze.

How can you tell if a clinic is doing this? They will have data from their patients that they have collected and reported, usually on an annual basis. Why is it important to see that clinic's data? A procedure like this may produce very different results in a different doctor's hands. In addition, the clinic will be able to tell you exactly how it collects its data, who collects it, how often, and so on. For example, a proper treatment registry collects data at set time points like one month, three months, six months, one year, two years, three years, and so on. If all you get is a call from a nurse, like you would after any common surgery, then this isn't nearly enough.

Guidance of the Injection

How we deliver stem cells as part of Interventional Orthopedics makes a big difference. While delivery into an arm vein (IV) is attractive because of the low level of expertise needed to deliver cells, studies have consistently shown that adult stem cells delivered in this fashion are trapped in the lungs (pulmonary first-pass effect). Of even more concern is a study showing that for patients considering the use of stem cells to treat central nervous system (CNS) disorders, only about 1 in 200,000 cells injected via an IV route reaches the brain and central nervous system (1.5- 3.7% made it past the lungs, 0.295% made it to the carotid artery, and 0.0005% made it past the blood-brain barrier into the brain). At this point, until these pulmonary first-pass issues are worked out, credible stem cell delivery is local. This means placing cells directly into the tissue or into the arterial circulation that directly supplies the tissue. In addition, based on our clinical experience, for orthopedic applications (and likely for others), it's hyperlocal, meaning that placement of cells into one part of the joint may provide results; whereas, nonspecific placement in the joint may provide fewer results. This means imaging guidance to place cells into joints is very important.

In addition, please note that the skills needed to place cells into very specific areas using an X-ray (fluoroscopy)- or ultrasound-guided injection are not common. For example, fewer than 1% of orthopedic surgeons have these advanced skills. In addition, while pain management physicians may have these X-ray–guidance skills in the spine, they usually have no ultrasound experience in how to place cells into peripheral joints, like the knee, hip, or shoulder. How can you tell if a doctor has this critical training? The Interventional Orthopedics Foundation (IOF) maintains a list on their website of accredited doctors (see www.interventionalorthopedics.org).

A Focus on Orthopedic Problems

Figuring out how to maximize the effects of stem cells is critical. Let me give you some examples. Early on in our experience, we added in the use of papers showing that it helped stem cells create more cartilage. We then had a natural experiment where we were able to compare patients who didn't have their cells exposed to this very low-dose medication versus those who did. The graph to the left shows how much better the patients who got the medication did, and as a result, this medication became a standard part of our protocol. This is just one example of how little things about how stem cell procedures are performed can make big differences.

As a result, it's not credible for a clinic to offer therapies for 10 different diseases that have little to do with each other. Credible clinics focus in on one or two body systems and perfect their treatment protocols. This is why we've kept our hyperfocus only on orthopedics and why we continue to do the basic science needed to improve our treatments. For a short video break, click on the Regenexx video link here.

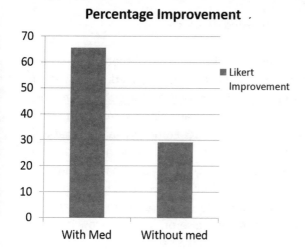

Percentage Improvement

Likert Improvement

(bar chart: With Med ≈ 65, Without med ≈ 29)

Candidacy Grading

There is no medical procedure available (including stem cells) where all patients are great candidates and expected to do well. Over the last almost decade that we have been offering stem cell treatments, we have graded patients with regard to candidacy. These good, fair, or poor candidate grades have literally dissuaded thousands of patients who were considered less-than-stellar candidates from undergoing the procedure. Several years ago, after we had enough outcome data on knee patients, we lifted those grades (for most patients) as the statistical analysis didn't show that more severe arthritis patients did any worse than patients with mild arthritis.

So, if you attend a seminar, ask the presenter who is a good or a poor candidate for this procedure? If he or she claims that the procedure works in everyone or that there is no such thing as a poor candidate, you should run. As no medical procedure ever devised works in all patients, and that includes stem cell therapy.

Also, if you get an evaluation by a clinic, ask about your candidacy. Is it good, fair, or poor, and why? Is anyone considered a poor candidate? For example, I can tell you that based on our existing registry data, if you have hip arthritis and are <u>over the age of 55, our data shows that you're less likely to do as well as someone who is younger</u>.

Published Research

In any new procedure, research should be published as the data becomes mature enough. We have always prided ourselves in <u>submitting our data to peer-reviewed journals for publication</u>. This takes an immense amount of work, as any single publication often goes back and forth for months to a year before it's in a form that will appease reviewers. So, ask if the clinic has research that they've published. Be careful here as this is a prime area for bait and switch; I've seen websites from clinics that show research that has nothing to do with the stem cell type or procedure they're using. For example, showing research done by someone else on bone-marrow-isolated mesenchymal stem cells when the clinic uses fat stromal vascular fraction (an apples-to-oranges comparison). This also happens when a clinic uses bone marrow. For example, I've seen clinics use my published research on their websites even when they don't use our proprietary procedure. How is that supposed to work? That's like saying someone published research on apples but the clinic uses oranges!

So, make sure you ask the following: *Where is your data on what **you** do? Where are publications I can find with **your name** on them*? Ninety-nine percent of the time, you'll find that the clinic has no such published data.

A Customized Approach to the Processing of Your Tissue

Every patient is unique, yet many clinics use automated one-size-fits-all machines to process tissue because the capital and time investment is **much less**. Most of these machines treat every sample as if it were the same, yet every sample is really quite different. Hence, what comes out of the machine is often not processed based on the individual characteristics of that tissue, so the stem cell yields are compromised. In addition, for bone marrow, all commercially available machines on the market today discard valuable stem cells that the Regenexx-SD procedure retains. Ask the clinic if they process your tissue by hand or if they use a small bedside machine that will treat you like a number rather than an individual.

A Clinical Training and Certification Program for Affiliates

There's a saying in medical training: "See one, do one, teach one." Regrettably, it refers to the practice of physicians often having very little experience or training before working on patients. The stem cell "wild west" exemplifies this problem.

Let me give you a real-world example. A few years back, I met a physician at a conference who was using bone marrow stem cells. He was describing his cell harvest technique from the back of the hip and mentioned that he took 100 cc of bone marrow from one site. I stopped him and asked who had taught him to do it that way? It turns out that a physician who visited our clinic (and was never trained by us) in 2007 had taught him this was the correct method. In fact, what that physician had seen was us taking 6–8 much smaller-volume samples because our own research and that of others had shown this technique dramatically increased the number of stem cells in the sample. The doctor who had visited simply didn't know why we were taking so much time to get so many samples, and he simplified the technique to a single high-volume sample. In the process, he also dramatically reduced the number of stem cells. He then went out and taught this modified technique to hundreds of physicians!

As a result, the Regenexx Network of physicians (location map to the right, click link above for specific provider information), whom we have officially trained, is the only stem cell provider network in the

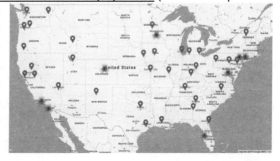

world with an extensive and mandatory clinical training program. First, rather than taking any willing provider, we turn down more physicians who want to join than we accept. Why? First, because they don't have the right skills to practice interventional orthopedics. Second, the few providers we do accept are extensively trained here in Colorado. This includes a **core skills checklist** of procedures they must know. In addition, treatment of any area (e.g., shoulder) has both a didactic education and hands-on demonstration of skills in a cadaver lab. This training goes through the nonprofit Interventional Orthopedics Foundation (IOF).

Regenexx Network physicians use the platelet procedures (Regenexx-PL and Regenexx-SCP) and same-day stem cell procedures (Regenexx-SD) and have in-house processing labs so they can customize the tissue processing to meet the needs of your sample. They also are part of our treatment registry. This means the outcomes we report include our own data plus the results obtained by our network providers.

I hope this detour into picking out the wheat from the stem cell chaff was helpful. Now let's explore why we believe many traditional drug approaches to joint arthritis, ligament/tendon tears, or spine diseases have problems. We'll also explore what alternative things you can do to help your ailing body.

Traditional Orthopedic Approaches

Let's explore some common traditional treatment approaches that may adversely impact how you respond to the newer biologic therapies, like platelets and stem cells. For example, steroids are commonly injected into joints, and patients are often prescribed nonsteroidal anti-inflammatory drugs (NSAIDs). Is this a good idea? Regrettably, the research of the past decade is increasingly showing that not only are many of these approaches ineffective, but some actually make the problems worse. Let's explore these a bit.

The Opposite of Healing: Apoptosis (Steroid Shots Are Bad News!)

What's the opposite of healing? Causing apoptosis, or

preprogrammed cell death without any ability to heal. For many years, doctors have injected <u>high-dose steroids</u> because they quickly bring down swelling and make the area feel better. <u>However, study after study continues to show that these drugs, when used at the high doses that physicians often inject (milligrams), cause local preprogrammed cell death (apoptosis)</u>. While causing a little cell injury is not necessarily a bad thing (as discussed above), steroids work by taking away the local repair response (<u>inflammation and swelling</u>) as well, and so you're left with an injured area that can't repair itself.

Doesn't the body use steroids? Yes, your body can release natural steroids into an area where the inflammation dial may be turned up too high, which turns down that inflammation dial just a smidge. How much is too much steroid? While <u>the milligrams</u> of steroid

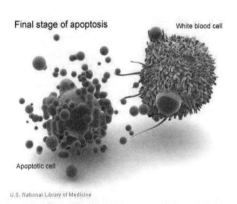

Final stage of apoptosis

White blood cell

Apoptotic cell

U.S. National Library of Medicine

commonly injected by doctors might not seem like much, it's about 100,000–1,000,000 times more steroid than your body would expect to see in the area. As an example, if the amount your body uses to control joint swelling is the height of a matchbook (<u>nanogram range</u>), the amount most doctors have been taught to inject is the height of the Empire State Building (milligram range)! Or, as I like to tell patients, if we inject the much smaller nanogram dose, we're putting in a thumbtack with a ball peen hammer, but if we inject the much larger milligram dose, it's like putting in the same thumbtack with a sledgehammer. If you use the ball peen hammer, there won't be much collateral damage, but using the sledgehammer is bound to create problems. Why don't we see more doctors injecting the smaller physiologic doses? For one reason, they just aren't commercially available in those dose ranges. Steroids for injection bought from a medical supply company come only in the much bigger milligram ranges. Despite injecting the much smaller doses, we usually see the same results (decreased swelling). <u>In addition,</u>

research has shown that these smaller doses can increase the good growth factors in a joint associated with repair.

Don't I Urgently Need to Get Rid of Inflammation?

The RICE approach in orthopedics has become widespread. The concept is to get rid of inflammation through rest, ice, compression, and elevation. But is getting rid of the inflammation always the best plan?

Inflammation—you've likely heard the term in a negative way. Inflammation means swelling. You've likely heard that too much inflammation in our arteries may be the cause of heart disease. You mayhave heard of a rare syndrome where too much inflammation after a leg or arm injury can cause serious problems (i.e., compartment syndrome, where out-of-control swelling in a confined space can lead to severe injury). All of this is true, but for this chapter, you have to understand that like anything, there is also a good side to inflammation. Without inflammation, we would never heal ourselves.

Maybe you've had a chronically swollen joint or seen people with joints that swell. The reaction from modern medicine has been to inject high- dose steroids into these joints. As stated above, since high-dose steroids are potent at reducing inflammation, this may at first seem to help. However, these ultra-high-dose drugs also destroy the natural repair response. So, we now have a joint that no longer swells but also has no ability to heal itself.

Why does a joint stay swollen? Swelling is the result of your body marshaling the troops to heal an area. All of the cell types needed to build new tissue are in the swollen area: cells to clean up the damaged tissue (macrophages), cells to recognize any foreign material and deactivate invaders (white blood cells), and stem cells to act as general contractors in managing the repair response (mesenchymal stem cells). However, your body will keep throwing inflammation (swelling) at the area if the right signal isn't received from the newly formed repair tissue. As discussed above, if there aren't enough stem cells to complete the construction project, the

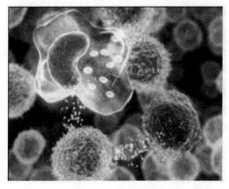

"done" signal may never be received.

An easy way to think about swelling is that it's like the heat in the oven that's used to bake a cake. After all, the term "inflammation" incorporates the Greek for the word for flame. When an area stays swollen and chronically inflamed, it's like low-level oven heat. If you place cake batter in a 200-degree oven, you don't end up with a baked cake but with dried out mush. Why? The chemical reaction that "bakes" the cake needs higher heat, or, said another way, to be more "inflamed." Turn up the oven to 400 degrees and you get a cake. The same holds true for a chronically swollen joint. The low heat of chronic inflammation isn't enough to repair the tissue, so the joint stays swollen. However, using the microinjury or platelet techniques above, we can "turn up the heat" and use much higher-level healing inflammation to heal the tissue (or bake the cake). The same can happen when we add stem cells, which can also help to complete the repair job.

So, in summary, inflammation isn't usually a bad thing in orthopedic applications. Swelling is necessary to heal. Doing things to get rid of swelling (the rest, ice, compression, elevation—or RICE—mantra) or using anti-inflammatory drugs may have their place in certain rare circumstances to prevent things like compartment syndromes. However, in Orthopedics 2.0, the use of drugs like high-dose steroids and NSAIDs (Motrin, ibuprofen, aspirin, Aleve, or other nonsteroidal anti-inflammatory drugs) to halt the healing inflammatory response is generally considered a bad idea.

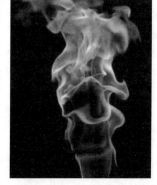

Getting Rid of the Steroids in Epidurals

Epidural steroid shots have become the de facto standard of care for patients with a pinched spinal nerve causing pain. This treatment involves injecting a high-dose steroid around the irritated nerve, usually using X-ray guidance to ensure accurate placement. However, steroid epidurals have been in the press lately for their negative side effects. In one study, <u>middle-aged and older women lost huge amounts of bone with each steroid epidural</u>. In another, <u>the part of the brain that reacts to stress</u> and various important hormones was knocked off-line for three weeks with each injection. Why? The amount of steroids in these shots is massive compared to what the body is used to seeing (more on this later in the "Neuromuscular" chapter). As a result, we have switched most of our epidural patients over to using platelet lysate instead of these high-dose toxic steroids. See this link for an infographic that goes over our registry data showing that <u>PL epidurals (Regenexx-PL-Disc) produce a better and more robust treatment outcome than steroid epidurals.</u>

Our licensees outside the United States also use various activated, incubated platelet supernatants or next-generation PRP. Think of these as PRP 2.0. To make these next-generation solutions, the lab starts with PRP, activates it with various natural substances, and <u>incubates</u> the platelets for several hours to several days. During this time the platelets are directed to produce certain natural growth factors that are important in specific types of healing. We then take that soup of natural growth factors and use that instead of PRP. For example, we can inject a solution that is rich in the <u>growth factor TGF-beta</u> (good at healing cartilage) by instructing the patient's platelets to produce more of that natural substance.

Should I Take Anti-inflammatory Pills to Help My Joints?
Medications That Adversely Impact Regenerative Orthopedics

Anti-inflammatory drugs have become a mainstay of orthopedic and musculoskeletal care. While we have discussed steroid medications, what about nonsteroidal anti-inflammatory drugs (NSAIDs)? These are medications that block the pathways for inflammation, with most of them, the COX (<u>cyclooxygenase</u>) pathway. COX drugs help control swelling, but they also cause stomach ulcers by inhibiting the enzyme that helps to protect the stomach wall. Just how dangerous are these drugs? Moore, in 2002, published that the estimated risk of death due to bleeding stomach ulcer when taking NSAIDs for more than 60 days was 1 in 1,200! While this represents only a small number of people who are very sensitive to this drug class, the overall numbers are concerning. As a result of these inherent dangers, newer drugs were designed to work against COX-2 rather than COX-1 (the latter being more responsible for protection of the stomach wall), but these drugs had a new set of side effects. These drugs (like Vioxx, Bextra, and Celebrex) all come with an enhanced cardiovascular risk (risk of sudden death by heart attack).

How do NSAIDs impact healing? Well, from a 50,000-foot view, inflammation is needed to heal, so blocking inflammation may inhibit healing. Sure enough, NSAID drugs, like Motrin and others, have been shown to delay healing. While most of this research has focused on fracture healing, we keep patients undergoing regenerative medicine treatments off these drugs. Other drugs are also notable for causing musculoskeletal problems. The antibiotic drug class that includes Cipro (quinalones) has been shown to lead to tendon ruptures. Heartburn drugs, like Nexium, have also been linked to hip fracture risk. Cholesterol drugs have been known to cause pain and harm muscles. Many commonly used drugs can adversely impact regenerative medicine healing. Our own cell-culture data implicates cholesterol and certain blood pressure drugs as causing problems with mesenchymal stem cell growth in culture.

If Most Drugs Are Bad News, What Else Can I Do?

Can you change your lifestyle to protect your joints? The answer is likely yes. I would break this down into a few different categories: diet, exercise, supplements, prescription medications, and hormones.

Diet

Could what you're eating impact your joints? We know that patients with metabolic syndrome get more arthritis, independent of their weight. What's a metabolic syndrome? This is when you gain weight (usually in middle age, but it can happen earlier), participate in limited exercise, and start to get high blood pressure. This happens because of a combination of genes, low activity levels, and a sugar/starch-based diet. Basically, excessive sugar and carbohydrate consumption leads to spikes in insulin, which eventually makes the pancreas less sensitive to insulin causing more to be produced. This "hyperinsulinism" leads to a state where insulin is always present, and this hormone is a potent blocker of fat breakdown and facilitator of fat production. All of this not only causes weight gain but also unstable blood sugar, which leads to bad chemicals that can break down cartilage. How do you fix it? Well, since you can't change your genes, you need to change your diet. If you want an instruction manual on how to eat, get one of the diet books, like Atkins, The Zone, The South Beach Diet, or The Paleo Diet, that focuses on weight loss through less sugar and carbs.

How do you know if you have better blood sugar control and, hence, are doing better protecting your cartilage? There are two tests, one that you can do at home and one that requires a doctor's visit. The first is what I call the "Dark Chocolate Test." Before you start on this diet, you'll likely think that a 70% dark chocolate bar tastes pretty bad or at least bitter. This is because you have set the level of sugar detection for your taste buds way too high by eating too much sugar and starch. However, once you are on a low-carb diet for a few months, the 70% should taste sweet. Next, try 80%. It should taste *OK* if you're a real low-carb superstar. If it doesn't, be stricter with your sugar intake. When you're done with your sugar transformation, an 85% bar will taste just fine, and that piece of birthday cake will be disgustingly sweet!

The doctor's office test is called an HbA1c serum level. This is a measure of changes to red blood cells in the presence of high blood sugar levels.   It can take a few months to change, so get it tested a few months into a diet. While your doctor may tell you that anything below a 6.0 is fine, it's really not. You want yours well below 5.6, and for maximum protection, it should be below 5.1. Remember, tracking this number takes patience! As your blood sugar control improves as you eat fewer carbs, this number may take many months to drop all the way to its nadir.

For more information on the right "stem cell" healthy diet, see Dr. Pitts's book *Nutrition 2.0* (click on the book cover to receive a free copy of this book).

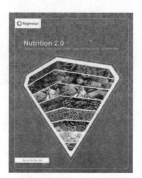

Exercise

First, what are "normal" levels of exercise for cartilage protection? Second, does pounding exercise, like running, destroy joints?
We Americans and others who live in first-world countries have become very accustomed to low exercise levels. My favorite candidacy review that I have ever performed was when I asked the personal physician of a Middle Eastern woman, who was a member of the royal family, whether the woman got much exercise. I was promptly told that the royal family took cars and a security detail to go around the block! While this is an extreme example, it gets the point across: we have lowered our expectations for exercise so much that we no longer know what our bodies were designed to do. Another example is the health club across the street from our office. I see people in there working out as if they are the walking dead, strolling along on an elliptical machine as if it were a Sunday stroll and not their half hour to work their body hard.

What our ancestors considered everyday activity, most of us would consider our toughest exercise day. Think about this for a moment. You wake up and haul 100 pounds of water a half mile from the river to your home. You then chop wood with a 30-pound iron axe for an hour. Then you get to walk/run 20 miles while you hunt the big game that will keep your family fed for the next week. You get the picture.

So, what is "normal activity" for our conversation on "Living 2.0"? It's 30–60 minutes of exercise so intense that having a normal conversation is very hard. This is performed five to six days a week and combined with weight lifting. In addition, my definition of weight lifting is absolutely not what I see in the gym across the street. Its 6–12 reps of whatever weight causes your muscles to fail by the 6th to 12th repetition. So, if its biceps curls, pick up the weight that will cause your biceps to stop working by the end of the set. Then do this twice more as a minimum biceps workout. Why am I pushing the weights so hard? <u>Because elderly weight lifters have muscles that at the cellular level look more like younger people than their old sedentary counterparts</u>. In addition, <u>exercise increases the stem cells in your muscles</u>.

What if pain prevents you from getting to this level? Well, that's why you're reading this book. Our goal is to use regenerative therapies, diet, exercise, and specialized therapies to keep you this active well into your 70s and beyond.

How about pounding exercise, like running? Is this good or bad for my joints? Regrettably, this <u>cartilage research is still all over the map</u>. Some studies have shown that running is protective to knee cartilage while others have shown it's destructive. In the meantime, like anything else, everything in moderation, or get a good doctor! By this, I mean that the ideal workout mixes up lots of activities, which might include running.

For more information on how to dial in your exercise to improve your stem cell health, see Dr. Williams's book *Exercise 2.0*.

Supplements

One of the most frequent questions I get asked by prospective stem cell patients is what supplements they should take to help their chances of success. While from looking at the ads on the Internet, this would appear to be a very simple question, it's actually quite complex. The issue is that while some supplements have been tested with cartilage cells, we have very few that have been tested with stem cells.

What I can say is mostly from tests with either cartilage cells or early studies in patients where objective measures of cartilage health are used (not stem cells).

- **Glucosamine** is a very common supplement that can be derived from many sources. It's basically a cartilage building block, and there's a bunch of research showing it helps cartilage. See article 1, article 2, and article 3.

• **Chondroitin** is the cousin of glucosamine and another common cartilage building block supplement. Many studies also show it helps cartilage. See article 1 and article 2.

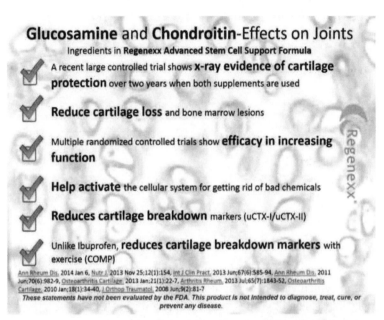

Glucosamine and Chondroitin-Effects on Joints
Ingredients in Regenexx Advanced Stem Cell Support Formula

✓ A recent large controlled trial shows **x-ray evidence of cartilage protection** over two years when both supplements are used

✓ **Reduce cartilage loss** and bone marrow lesions

✓ Multiple randomized controlled trials show **efficacy in increasing function**

✓ **Help activate** the cellular system for getting rid of bad chemicals

✓ **Reduces cartilage breakdown** markers (uCTX-I/uCTX-II)

✓ Unlike Ibuprofen, **reduces cartilage breakdown markers** with exercise (COMP)

Ann Rheum Dis. 2014 Jan 6. Nutr J. 2013 Nov 25;12(1):154. Int J Clin Pract. 2013 Jun;67(6):585-94. Ann Rheum Dis. 2011 Jun;70(6):982-9. Osteoarthritis Cartilage. 2013 Jan;21(1):22-7. Arthritis Rheum. 2013 Jul;65(7):1843-52. Osteoarthritis Cartilage. 2010 Jan;18(1):34-40. J Orthop Traumatol. 2008 Jun;9(2):81-7
These statements have not been evaluated by the FDA. This product is not intended to diagnose, treat, cure, or prevent any disease.

• **Fish Oil** is a supplement that is taken widely, but poorly understood by most who take it. While this is an important source of omega-3 fatty acids that can help reduce swelling, and there's some evidence that it may help preserve cartilage, most people take way too little to see these effects. First, you need to make sure your fish oil isn't oxidized. So, if your fish oil smells fishy, ditch it and get a better brand. Second, if you pop a few pills that you bought in a grocery store with the label "Fish Oil," you're taking way under the dosage associated with big health benefits (the amounts that Greenland Eskimos consume). Using that math, it would take 20-30 pills per day of these garden variety capsules to match this amount. An easier way to take more omega-3s is to buy concentrated EPA/EFA brands. This is about 3,000-6,000 mg of omega-3 fatty acids per day. More on all of this at this link.

- **Curcumin** is an extract from the Indian spice turmeric. <u>The research looks promising that it's an anti-inflammatory and may help preserve cartilage.</u> In fact, <u>a recent study shows that it's as good as Motrin for pain and swelling</u>. It also seems to work better when combined with other supplements like resveratrol.

How does the supplement Curcumin stack up against NSAID drugs?

   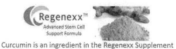

Over the counter and prescription NSAID Drugs	Curcumin is an ingredient in the Regenexx Supplement
✓ Positive effects in arthritis	✓ Positive effects in arthritis
✗ Reduces bone healing and hurts the ability of stem cells to repair cartilage	✓ Enhances healing and helps the ability of stem cells to repair cartilage (in-vitro)
✗ Increases systemic inflammatory markers	✓ Decreases systemic inflammation
✗ Increases oxidative stress	✓ Anti-oxidant
✗ Increases deadly heart attack risk by 200-300%	✓ Reduces CRP, a marker associated with elevated heart risk

These statements have not been evaluated by the FDA. This product is not intended to diagnose, treat, cure, or prevent any disease.
ScientificWorldJournal. 2014 Feb 11:2014:898361. J Infect Dis. 1991 Jan:163(1):89-95. Chem Biol Interact. 2012 Jul 30;199(1):15-28, Int Immunopharmacol. 2014 Mar 24, J Orthop Res. 2013 Feb;31(2):235-42 Arthritis Res Ther. 2010;12(4):R127. doi: 10.1186/ar3065. Tissue Eng Part A. 2013 Apr;19(7-8):1039-46., Clin Interv Aging. 2014 Mar 20;9:451-8, Phytother Res. 2013 Aug 7

- **Resveratrol** is a powerful antioxidant and activator of the SIRT1 gene which has been associated with longevity. It's found principally in the skin of grapes, and it's thought to be one reason the French suffer fewer cardiac events. Apparently, all of that red wine is loaded with resveratrol! <u>It also seems to help poor blood sugar control. That middle-aged paunch caused by declining insulin control can also eat up cartilage</u>, so resveratrol may protect joints.

There are literally a hundred other supplements touted as good for arthritis. However, our patients also want supplements that will help their stem cells, yet little stem cell research exists with supplements, which is why we had to create our own.

At first, I thought this would be a quick two to three-month project of testing stem cells with supplements to see how they grew. As we got further into this project of determining which supplements were the best at stimulating stem cells to grow more cartilage, the science got more and more complex. We learned we needed to look at the following:

> How the stem cells from the bone marrow of different ages of donors responded to different supplements. Most studies in this area choose young stem cells by default since samples are often bought through a science company or taken from grad students. Yet older stem cells are different and need to be tested alongside younger cells. In addition, the stem cells from arthritis patients are likely different, and few twentysomething grad students have arthritis. As a result, we took all of our cells from real arthritis patients.

> How the stem cells grew when exposed to supplements. This is not so easy as many supplements are digested into different forms before they reach the bloodstream, so we tested these forms as well.

> How well the stem cells produced cartilage components when exposed to various supplements. To do this, we needed to look at the cells as they produced these cartilage-building blocks with quantitative fluorescent microscopy. To the right is an example of what this looks like, with the bright areas representing the amount of cartilage components—collagen 2, aggrecan, and SOX9—being produced by the cells.

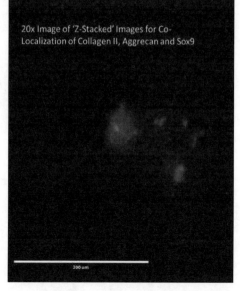

20x Image of 'Z-Stacked' Images for Co-Localization of Collagen II, Aggrecan and Sox9

200 um

> How well these supplements were able to support the overall robustness of the cells. A cell can look great in culture, grow well, and produce cartilage, but how healthy is it when stressed? In medicine, an example is the stress test for the heart. While someone might appear healthy, when they're

pushed to the limit on a treadmill, their heart can show signs of trouble. We did the same thing for cells by adding in common bad chemicals found in arthritic joints that beat up cells like IL-6 and then seeing if the supplements helped the cells recover better.

➢ Determining the sourcing. Most supplements come from many different sources. As an example, glucosamine can be extracted from any number of shellfish sources, pig parts, or cow parts. Is one of these better than the other at helping human stem cells?

➢

In the end, after a year of testing, we produced a supplement we could hang our hat on: Regenexx Advanced Stem Cell Support Formula. One that was based on basic research that we felt represented what we were trying to accomplish in patients. While every other supplement you can buy is merely put together based on snippets of data taken from unrelated lab research done by others, ours was a coordinated and costly plan to find the best ingredients for our patients. Click on the video link below to see a short animation on the Regenexx Supplement.

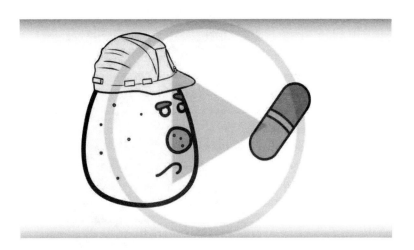

Prescription Medications

When we first began culturing cells in 2006, we were surprised to find that some patients' stem cells wouldn't grow well. After a few culture failures, we decided to try and isolate the problem, and after much trial and error, we were surprised to learn that the culprit was usually a prescription medication. For example, when we would stop the patient's medication and take new cells and reculture them, the stem cells would grow fine. We could also get the cells to grow fine when we exposed them to the serum of another person who wasn't on the drug (for research purposes only). This convinced us that many prescription medications are toxic to stem cells.

What should you avoid? Likely, the most surprising thing we encountered was that America's wonder drug, cholesterol medications known as statins, seemed toxic to stem cells. I would take a minute to read about the limited efficacy of these drugs if you're on them, but only make any decisions to stop the drug after consulting your primary care physician. Other drugs that were problems included NSAIDs like ibuprofen, Motrin, Aleve, and Celebrex. Given that NSAID drugs carry significant cardiac risks, not taking these drugs makes sense. We have found fish oil makes a great alternative anti-inflammatory, and research supports this effect. Other problem drugs include ACE inhibitor blood pressure medications that are usually taken to combat hypertension due to metabolic syndrome. Rather than take these drugs, increase activities and cut the carbs to control your blood pressure. Finally, steroid anti-inflammatories are also a big concern, as they are toxic to many different cell types, including stem cells.

Hormones

We take our hormonal mix for granted, a little like the fact that our heart beats more than 100,000 times a day. Yet if you're trying to control your weight and stem cells, these hormones can play a critical role as you age. For example, serum taken from women after menopause (when many hormones are no longer produced) directs stem cells that should turn to bone to turn into fat instead. For men, testosterone levels decline as we age. Yet testosterone can activate stem cells to produce more muscle and less fat. While the jury is still out on the effects of sex hormones on stem cells, in men it's pretty clear that supplementing these hormones in middle-aged and elderly patients can help overall body composition, reducing fat and increasing lean muscle mass and likely improving heart health. The same has been shown for women. On the other hand, the willy-nilly prescribing of testosterone in men, without strict monitoring, may be linked to an increase in heart attacks.

Should you supplement your hormones? This is a personal decision. In my experience, it makes it much easier to keep the pounds off and activity levels high as we age. On the flip side, for men, urologists have been concerned that testosterone may cause prostate cancer. However, newer research suggests this likely isn't the case. In addition, without strict monitoring, the excess production of blood cells may be the cause of blood clots that can cause heart attacks. For women, the Women's Health Initiative study suggested that estrogen pills could cause cancer, yet the study authors have since stated that the press misinterpreted their results. They now recommend hormone therapy for younger women just after menopause.

My Own Living 2.0 Story

When I was 37, I was at the low point of my personal health. My wife and I had just gone through the trauma of having premature twins, and my exercise was sparse while my sleep was nonexistent. My weight had ballooned such that my waist had gone from a 32 while in residency to a 42. Just jumping onto our high bed made my heart race. I was an early heart attack waiting to happen. It took a decade to completely climb out of the hole I dug, and I've learned quite a few things. Had I known these at 37, I could have been in perfect shape by 40!

What did I learn along the way?

➢ **Carbs are key**. While for my wife's genetics, carbs aren't important, for me they are everything. I spent years on fad diets, trying to prevent my waist from ballooning and avoiding any type of shopping for pants (as that meant admitting that I could no longer fit into a size 40), none of which worked. In the end, it was understanding that limiting my sugars and starchy carbs was the answer. However, that got me only part of the way there.

➢ **What the term "workout" means**. Like I have said, I see people working out at the gym like they're the walking dead, and I understand that once that was me. It wasn't until I got a personal trainer that I finally understood what working out was all about. My trainer worked me like a dog, and the harder he pushed the more I wanted. It took a few years with a trainer to understand that to stay in good shape in middle age for most of us requires working very hard. An example is the INSANITY workouts. For most of those 30–40 minutes, the exercise is tough enough that holding a conversation is difficult—you're simply pushing too hard. A kinder and gentler approach that starts slow and builds (by the same trainer) is FOCUS T25. The same applies with weights, which should be a cardio workout as well. If you're not huffing and puffing while you quickly move from one weight station to the next, you're not hitting it hard enough.

When I finally figured this out, my weight went down again. But there was still one more piece.

➢ **Hormonal control** is a problem for middle-aged men and women. I spent many years being asked to lecture to doctors involved in age-management medicine as many are very interested in stem cells. I would sit through the lectures before and after mine, which were about supplementing hormones in middle-aged and elderly men and women. I have to say that at first, I thought these doctors were a bit nuts. Was this really necessary? After a few years of seeing countless lecturers review the science, I was convinced that I had to be my own guinea pig. In 2010, I worked with a Denver-based age-management specialist to check my testosterone levels. They were dismally low, so I started testosterone therapy. The final piece of the puzzle clicked into place for me. Much of the extra weight that I had been carrying melted off as I already had the diet and exercise piece under good control. Unlike the recent rush to prescribe testosterone to everyone with "Low T," this program is carefully monitored. Which brings me to the last part.

➢ **Proactive injury management is important**. You can't help but get injured from time to time if you're hitting exercise hard enough to stay active as you age. I constantly look at my joint stability, levels of nerve irritation, muscular firing, and body symmetry—just as I describe in this book. All of this is to try and prevent injuries or catch problems when they're early. Since supplementing testosterone pushes my blood hematocrit up (the number of red blood cells), I put those extra blood cells to good use. Once every two to three months, I have blood taken to reduce my hematocrit and to fuel the Regenexx-SCP and Regenexx-PL procedures. I proactively have small issues treated with these regenerative cocktails. As an example, my right knee, left shoulder AC joint, right elbow, and low back are common problem areas for me. These aren't disabling problems but are areas of constant irritation—all likely related to wear and tear and declining stem cell activity as I age. So, I have my colleagues give these areas an "espresso shot" of my own healing blood platelets.

The conclusion? For me, controlling my weight, staying off prescription drugs, and staying active requires four key elements: diet, exercise, hormones, and early injury detection and management.

Chapter 4: Symmetry

STABILITY
The ability of a joint to tightly move as it was designed without extra motions that might hurt the joint.

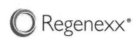

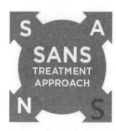

S   A
SANS
TREATMENT
APPROACH
N   S

www.regenexx.com

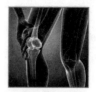

ARTICULATION
The health of the joints. Shock-absorbing tissues like cartilage; spacer tissue such as meniscus; or stabilizing tissues such as labrum can be damaged.

NEUROMUSCULAR
The nerves drive the muscles. Nerves that are irritated or compressed cause pain and may be less able to promote muscles to properly fire.

SYMMETRY
The left/right and front/back balance of the body. When the body is asymmetrical, certain parts get injured or wear out faster.

"True freedom is where an individual's thoughts and actions are in alignment with that which is true, correct, and of honor—no matter the personal price."
Bryant H. McGill

Symmetry

In most patients, there's usually more joint damage on one side than the other. Why? If someone has a genetic predisposition to arthritis and this is the only factor causing the joints to degenerate, shouldn't all joints be affected equally? In addition, osteoarthritis is more commonly seen first in the knees and hips and less often in the ankles and elbows. Why? Again, shouldn't we see all joints being impacted the same? The reason is clear: the wear and tear on our joints occurs unevenly, with some being impacted more than others or one side undergoing more wear than the other.

Why Should I Care About My Symmetry?

If you don't want to stay active and pain free as you age, then ignore this chapter. If you do want to stay active, then pay attention! Your body is designed to be symmetrical, and even slight amounts of extra force or motion, in any area, caused by an unbalanced body will cause problems. These may start small, but like a snowball rolling down hill, they become bigger and bigger with time.

Reducing the Wear and Tear

As already discussed, increasing healing ability is only one part of the Orthopedics 2.0 equation. The other half of this coin is reducing the

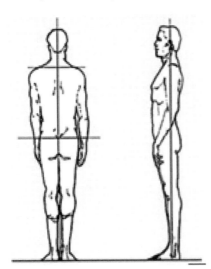

wear and tear forces that destroyed the joint in the first place. As an example, placing new tires on a car with bad alignment, without fixing the alignment, is guaranteed to quickly wear out the tires again. This issue is often ignored in our current quick-fix treatment methodology. I've seen hundreds of patients with a specific wear pattern, like on the right medial meniscus, where the most salient questions have never been asked: how did this knee get like this, and what are we going to do to ensure that it doesn't get this way again?

The reason the issue of specific wear-and-tear patterns is mostly ignored is that it's complex. Most physicians aren't trained to understand the biomechanics of the body. The few physical therapists or other providers who have spent years of extra study learning biomechanics are often too heavily incentivized by insurance companies to take the time needed to figure out why a part keeps failing.

Let's use a simple example to illustrate this concept. The skeleton on the right has been drawn with red force arrows going down from the hips. Let's say that for an unknown reason, slightly more force is applied to the right side (the thicker arrow) than the left side (the thinner arrow). We take thousands of steps a day. What happens to the extra forces on the right, and how does the body handle them? The right hip, knee, and ankle will all react. They will initially just shore up the bones, tendons, ligaments, cartilages, and muscles on that side. When this person is young, with many adult stem cells in these areas, he or she may not notice much. However, as the number of adult stem cells begins to decrease with aging, the damage due to wear and tear at some point will begin to overtake the repair ability of these tissues and react to the extra forces. These areas (the ones

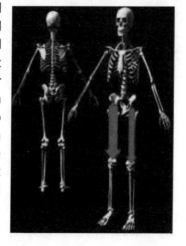

that are the most vulnerable) will begin to break down. If our only goal is to replace one of the right-sided joints with an artificial joint, that prosthesis may wear out a bit faster on that side, but this is likely not a huge issue. However, if we want to preserve that right-sided joint with Orthopedic 2.0-type procedures, we had better figure out why that joint is getting so much more wear and tear and correct that problem.

Take Five Minutes to Understand Your Symmetry

Patients are often surprised to find out that their body is no longer symmetrical. Others have noticed that a certain area has been getting tight for years. Either way, going through an intensive five-minute test of all major body joints, checking for symmetry, is well worth your time. Why? As discussed above, joints that are not equal in their side-to-side or front-to-back motion don't wear evenly. If you have any areas that are tight and not symmetrical and you don't figure out what's going on and fix these, you can bet arthritis is in your future if it's not already knocking at the door. In fact, symmetry is often the single biggest thing that you can work to fix that may either allow you to have an active older age or one plagued by problems and inactivity.

This is an 11-step test. You need to focus on whether you can attain the movement to the degree asked, whether the right and left are identical or different, whether the front and back is the same or different, and whether the tightness in the lettered areas is different on one side or the other. Realize the differences may be subtle, but important. In addition, pay attention to which movements cause pain and where. **If you're a patient of our clinic or a patient of a Regenexx Network physician, fill out the form in appendix A and bring it to your visit.**

If any movement causes significant pain, stop immediately and see a doctor. **If you think any of these motions may injure you, or you are prone to injuries with common or unusual movement, don't do this test, and, instead, see a physician.**

Step 1: Protracted Shoulder Check

Stand normally and place your hands together. Raise them over your head as shown. Move the hands as far back as they will go. Pay attention to whether the shoulders go back equally (you may want to have someone check, or do this in a mirror). Also pay attention to whether the front of the shoulders at points A and B are equally tight or if one of them is painful. You can also do this same maneuver lying flat on your back on a firm surface. In that case, your hands should touch the floor. If they don't, then both sides of your chest are too tight, or you may have problems with the range of motion of the large shoulder joint. This step checks your ability to abduct the shoulder and also checks the tightness in the pectoralis major and minor muscles along with the front and bottom of the shoulder capsule.

If this causes shoulder pain, you may have a shoulder impingement, a problem where the structures of the shoulder are getting pinched by poor movement patterns.

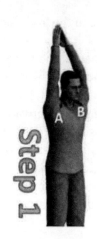

Step 2: Posterior Shoulder Check

Stand normally and place one hand behind your back. Raise it up as high as it will go. Both hands should be able to go at least to the middle of your upper back with the thumb just below the shoulder blades. Notice whether both sides can go equally as high and whether you have tightness in the back of the shoulder at points A and B. Is one side tighter than the other? This movement measures the tightness in the infraspinatus muscle as well as the back of the shoulder capsule.

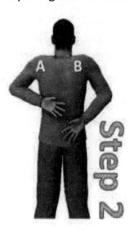

Patients who can't do this tend to develop overload on the back of the shoulder joint where they can develop labral tears. While many surgeons would just focus on the labral tear, the real focus should be on why this shoulder can't internally rotate!

Step 3: Neck Check

Very slowly and carefully roll your neck 360 degrees (only 180 is shown). Does this cause any pain at any point? Does it roll equally well to the front, side, and back? Is one side tighter than the other?

Patients who don't do well with going straight back or back and to the sides may have an arthritic or injured facet joint in the neck or a problem with lordosis (discussed later in this chapter). If bending to the side or forward is tough, you may have tightness in the postural muscles of the neck that hold the head up, like the levator scapula, upper trapezius, or cervical extensors. Finally, if one of the front muscles is tight, it could be the stenocleidomastoid, an important muscle that helps to turn the head. You may also notice that you can't hold your head back like this or that if feels out of control if you do.

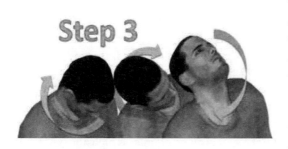

This is often caused by weakness in the deep neck flexors, like longus colli or longus capitis. Weakness in these deep neck flexor muscles can lead to chronic headaches. In the "Neuromuscular" chapter (next chapter), there's a strength and endurance test that also covers this issue.

Step 4: Cervical and Thoracic Rotation Check
While standing, place your hands on your chest, and turn your head all the way over your shoulder as far as it will go. Then follow through with a rotation of your upper back as far as it will go with your feet firmly planted (they shouldn't move). Do this on both sides.

Can you turn as far with your neck and your upper back on the left as on the right? Is there more tightness on one side of the neck, upper back, or lower back than on the other?

Patients who can't turn their neck may have a problem

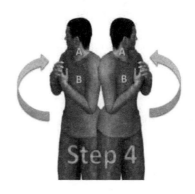

with the facet joints; whereas, patients who can't turn their upper back may have that issue or a problem with the normal motion of the rib cage, the rib attachments at the spine (called rib facets), or the thoracic spinal facet joints. In addition, chronic chest wall tightness on one or both sides may also limit the rotation of the upper back.

Step 5: Hip Rotation Check

Stand normally and place the toes of your feet together as shown. Make sure your feet are aligned and symmetrical—it's easy to cheat by placing one foot forward or back. Note whether both feet move inward equally (the motion is mostly coming from your hips). Also note the A and B points listed in the front 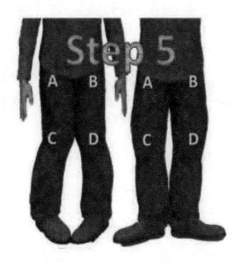 and back of the hips. Are these areas equally tight? Is one tighter than the other? Also note the C and D points—does any of this stress or hurt your knees or one knee? Now take your toes and rotate them out all the way. Again, be careful to make sure your feet are symmetrical (heels are together) as otherwise it's cheating.

If one hip has a very different range of motion (toes don't move as far in or out, and this seems to be due to tightness in the hip), this is very concerning. The hips tend to lose range of motion quickly and almost always after the onset of moderate or severe arthritis. I would advise you to get your hip checked immediately by your physician. If you already know you have a hip problem, this means that you have serious work to do. Unlike other joints, the hip has a very limited weight-bearing area (the part of the joint where it gets the most force). When the hip loses range of motion, and when arthritis is already present, the joint will put much more pressure on already worn areas, hastening cartilage loss. Getting hip range of motion back can be a challenge. In addition, patients with poor hip range of motion tend to have a less robust response to stem cell injections. As a result, there are procedures we can use to try and improve the hip range of motion through an injection that stretches the joint capsule.

Step 6: Lateral Hip and Back Check

Stand normally and reach to the side as shown. Go as far as you can, and note points A and B. Can you go as far on the right as you can on the left? Does one side of the lower back and/or outside hip feel tighter (point A or B)? Does that tightness extend down the side of the leg to the knee (points C and D)? This step measures the tightness in the opposite lateral lower and upper back muscles, like the quadratus lumborum and 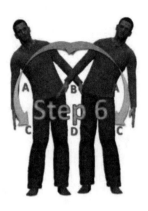 iliocostalis lumborum. It also measures the tightness of the opposite lateral hip muscles, like the tensor fascia latae and iliotibial band.

If you can't bend as much to one side, there may be tightness in these muscles or the spine. If you have pain that goes down the side of the hip and leg, you may have an SI joint problem with tightness in the iliotibial band or an S1 nerve problem in your back.

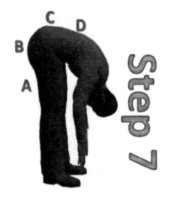

Step 7: Gluteal, Lumbar, and Thoracic Extensor Check

Bend forward all the way, and try and touch your toes. Do you get pain or severe tightness in one or both hamstrings (point A)? Is one side of your buttocks tighter than the other (point B)? Is your lower or upper back tight (points C and D)? Can you get within six inches of the floor? Does this cause pain or perhaps

122

tightness, numbness, or tingling in one or both legs? Is your belly in the way?

Patients who have difficulty getting close to the floor have significant tightness in hip flexion (which could be arthritis) or lower/upper back flexion (which could be disc disease or extensor muscle tightness). If one hamstring is always tight despite your best efforts to stretch it, it could actually be an irritated S1 nerve in your back despite the fact that your back doesn't hurt that much. Irritated nerves in your back can also cause one or both legs to get tingly in this position.

Step 8: Hip Flexor, Ankle Dorsiflexion, and Forefoot Check

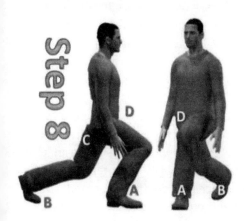

Perform a lunge as shown, getting as far down as you can, making sure you feel a good stretch in the front of the hip on the back leg. On that leg, bend your toes so that they meet the floor flat. On the other leg, flex the ankle as much as possible. For some people, getting a good stretch may involve placing the hands all the way down to the floor. Notice the front of the ankle of the forward leg, and compare that to the other side when you perform the opposite stretch (point A). Does the buttock on the front leg have the same side to side tightness? On the back leg, can you flex your toes (point B), or is this restricted on one side or painful? On the same leg, is the front of the hip (point D) equally tight on both sides, or is one side tighter? Can you get as low on each side?

Patients who have difficulty at point A (front of the ankle) may have ankle arthritis or a bone spur in the front of the tibiotalar joint, restricting dorsiflexion of the ankle. Patients with problems at B (toes) may have arthritis at the metatarsophalangeal (MTP) joints in the foot. <u>For the big and second toe, this can sometimes be related to long-standing low-back problems (even though you think your back is fine)</u>.

Patients with problems at C (buttocks) may have problems with hip flexion, indicating tight gluteal muscles or arthritis in the hip. Pain with this maneuver could also mean a labral tear in the front of the hip. Finally, if you have an issue at D (front of the hip), this could indicate a tight psoas muscle. This muscle goes from the front of the lumbar spine to the hip, so tightness here can be due to chronic low-back issues or trigger points in this muscle. Sometimes patients with psoas issues have trouble getting in and out of a low car.

Step 9: Knee-Extensor Mechanism Check

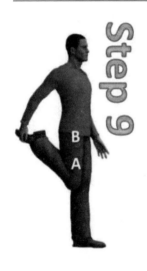

Stand normally and grab one foot with the same hand while bending the knee as shown. You may need to hold onto something. That's actually your first observation. If you can't easily balance like this (after a practice run), then you have significant low-back and hip-stability problems on the opposite side of the knee bend (see the <u>"Stability" chapter</u>). For the symmetry check, do the right and left knees bend equally? To really check this, make sure you stand straight while checking both sides. Does point A (quadriceps) feel the same on each side? How about the front of the hip (point B). Does either knee hurt in this position?

If you have less knee bending on either side, the simplest explanation is that you have trigger points in the quadriceps muscle (see next chapter). If the front of the hip is tight, you may have issues with the rectus femoris muscle. If the knee hurts, you may have a patellofemoral problem (an issue with the kneecap in its groove). Another common cause of asymmetry here is swelling in the knee joint due to chronic arthritis, which reduces the ability of the knee to flex.

Step 10: Adductor, Sartorius, and Gracilis Check

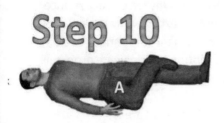

Lie on the floor and place one ankle over the opposite knee as shown. Next, try to get the bent knee as low to the floor as possible. Check both sides and see if they are equal in your ability to get the ankle high up on the opposite knee. See if point A (inside of the thigh) feels the same degree of tightness side to side? Can you get one bent knee farther toward the floor than the other?

Tightness in these muscles of the inside of the thigh are common in patients with chronic low-back conditions and sometimes can cause hip or inside-of-knee pain. In addition, patients with hip arthritis may notice a difference in flexibility from side to side.

Step 11: Lumbar and Thoracic Extension Check

Lie face down and prop up on your elbows, arching your back by lifting your head as high as possible and pushing your hips into the floor. Can you do this without pain? Does your lower back (point A) or upper back (point B) feel tight or hurt? Do you have pain or tightness at the back of the shoulder blades?

Patients who have tightness in the front of the hip and low back may have tight psoas muscles. Patients who have pain in their low back with this maneuver may have injured or arthritic low-back facet

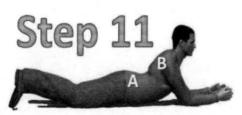

joints. If you have pain in one shoulder blade, there could be a problem in the joint between the shoulder blade and ribs or in the rib cage itself.

What do you do now with this information? If you have an area where your movement isn't normal, or there's a noticeable side to side difference in motion or tightness, there may be a few different causes. First, this needs to be looked at by a physician, physical therapist, or other musculoskeletal provider. Why? In our experience, asymmetrical motion is a leading cause of excessive wear-and-tear arthritis, so getting symmetrical and balanced motion back is absolutely critical. Second, the lack of motion may indicate problems in that joint that have yet to be addressed.

What are some common ways to treat these tight areas?

1.   Do simple stretches. The longest running stretching book on the market is Bob Anderson's. See this link for Amazon or this one for the basic stretches.

2.   Clear trigger points. When I discuss specific muscles above, these are your areas to target. Many times, there are knots in the muscles that when cleared will allow normal movement. The next chapter will focus more on ways to get rid of these trigger points.

3.   Repair irritated nerves. Sometimes an irritated nerve won't allow normal motion in an area, as a protective response for the nerve. This topic is dealt with in the next chapter.

4.   Treat joint arthritis. Sometimes an arthritic joint won't allow motion because bone spurs within the joint are blocking motion or the covering of the joint (the capsule) is too tight. For information on these issues, see the "Articulation" chapter.

Now That You Know You Have Problems, Let's Learn More About Symmetry

We'll start first with the spine, as your arms, legs, and head would be useless without an anchor point. This anchor is your spinal column. You might be saying, But I have a shoulder or knee problem. Why should I care about the spine? Because regardless of where you feel the pain, it's almost impossible for your spine not to be involved in some way.

A recent documentary on the tragedy of 9/11 provides a vivid example that may help bring this concept home. On one of the upper floors, many workers were trapped by a door to the stairs that wouldn't open. No matter how many large guys tried to ram it open, it wouldn't budge. It turns out that the violence of the airplane strike had twisted the spine of the building ever so slightly, and this compressed the doorframe against the door. These workers were eventually saved by a heroic building super who guessed accurately that kicking a hole in the drywall next to the doorframe might release the pressure on the door. Your spine is the same. Small issues here can cause large problems in your shoulders, arms, hands, hips, legs, ankles, or feet.

Lordosis in the Spine, or It's All About the Curves

<u>Lordosis</u> is the medical term for a front-back spinal curve. A healthy body in normal standing strives to use as little energy as possible. The

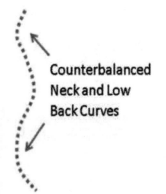

Counterbalanced Neck and Low Back Curves

diagram to the left shows how the neck and low-back curves are counterbalanced so that you can stand up straight with a minimal amount of effort.

Far too little attention has traditionally been placed on these curves, but the medical and surgical community is slowly changing their position on this important issue. <u>Researchers have completed clinical trials showing that rehabilitation efforts to restore these curves do produce positive clinical results</u>. Some spine surgeons now routinely take extra time and energy to restore or preserve the normal or natural spinal curve when performing fusions and disc replacements.

Why are these so important? First, it's all about energy consumption. A way to help you understand this is in the challenges facing modern robotics. A dream of robot designers has been to design an android robot that can cook and clean your house like a personal servant. The problem was that designing a robot that could really walk like a human turned out to be a huge engineering nightmare. However, when engineers solved that, <u>they soon realized that the human body</u>

had another secret. It uses very little energy to walk, whereas their robot was an energy hog, lasting only 30 minutes on battery power. Why? The body is designed to conserve energy in movement, and it all starts with the spinal curves. These finely tuned curves allow you to stand using almost no energy. Knock one out by causing straightening and it dramatically upsets the whole system. In addition, the wear and tear on certain structures changes dramatically as well.

How would you know if you have bad spinal curves? It can be found on your MRI or X-rays, but these issues aren't often identified by the

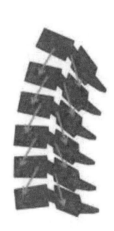

reading radiologist. It usually takes a doctor who's looking for these issues. Why is this big deal? It can fry your neck or back discs, leading to more bulges, tears, and herniations.

Each vertebra (spine bone) is built and oriented in such a way as to equally distribute forces between the front part (the disc) and the back part (the facet joints). This only happens when the normal spinal curves (lordosis) are present (see image on the left).

When the curve is lost (straight spine), the forces get distributed more toward the disc, which can cause it to get overloaded. We often see this on MRIs as swelling in the vertebra around the disc (which means the disc isn't capable of handling all of these forces, and they're getting distributed to the surrounding bone). The official medical term for this MRI finding is a "Modic change." Note the diagram to the right, which shows a loss of curve and a move of forces (large red arrows) to the front of the spine (disc).

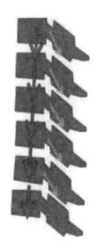

This loss of spine curve is a problem when considering stem cell therapy or any other type of regenerative procedure on the disc because while such a procedure might be able to help keep the disc from failing, the same forces that caused the disc to fail in the first place (loss of the spinal curve, placing too much pressure on the disc), will persist. So, we believe it's better to have the patient undergo therapy to restore the normal curve either before or during regenerative disc therapy.

What happens if the curve is too much? In that case, this is called a hyperlordosis (see figure on left), and the weight gets distributed too much to the facet joint. 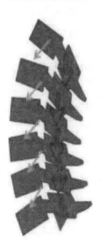 These little joints are about the size of your finger joints and live in pairs at the back of the spine. There are two at each spinal level, with one on the left and one on the right. They help to control motion, so that any specific vertebra can't get too far out of line. When they get overloaded by a big spinal curve, they can get arthritis much more quickly and show signs of wear, such as cysts and hypertrophy (the body will literally make them bigger to handle the extra weight). When these joints become bigger (arthritis), they can place pressure on the nearby exiting spinal nerves, and cause a new set of problems.

Forward Head, Kyphosis, and Lower Neck Joints

As discussed above, the spine is a delicately balanced machine where the neck and low-back curves are counterbalanced by the thoracic curve. As we age, our head and shoulders tend to hunch forward as shown on next page. As this happens, in order for us to see straight again, we crank our necks back farther. Because of this extra backward pressure on the neck, the facet joints in the bottom of the neck can be compressed, causing pain and more arthritis at those levels. While performing traditional facet injections into these aggravated joints can help, it does nothing to solve the excess loads on the area, so the pain just returns. This is a great example of how Orthopedics 2.0 differs from pain management. The pain management approach is to put steroid anti-

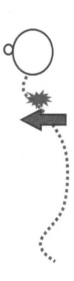

<u>inflammatories</u> into the joint to reduce pain. The Orthopedics 2.0 approach is to treat the joint (more likely with either low- dose anti-inflammatories or regenerative techniques), but also to work on getting weight off the joints by implementing a therapy regime that restores the proper curve, posture, or alignment.

Can Your Forward Head Cause Shoulder Arthritis?

What causes shoulder arthritis? If your shoulders have been aching as you age, you may want to pay attention. Are you in the early stages of shoulder arthritis? Is there something you can do to combat this arthritis and a forward head? Note the diagram above. When you're younger, your head and shoulders are straight and aligned with a perfectly balanced spine (neck curve points one-way, upper back curve balances it by pointing the other, and your low back curves back the other way). Note that the blowup of the side and front views of the normal shoulder on the left has the ball perfectly aligned in the socket. As you get older, your head and shoulders and spine begin to move forward (due to our habit of sitting in chairs). As this progress, the upper back part of the spine can become kyphotic (humpbacked). In fact, you may be noticing that you now have to catch yourself as it becomes more natural to be in that kyphotic (slouched) position.

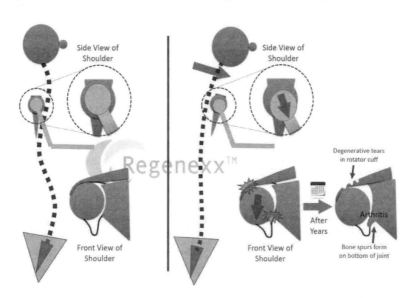

130

What does all of this have to do with your shoulders? As you become more kyphotic (see right above), your shoulders will begin to move forward. This has caused the ball of the shoulder joint to fall forward and down, out of the shallow socket. The new position now requires the rotator cuff (red in the front-shoulder blowup on the right above) to have to resist that new downward hanging force. In addition, it overstresses the top and bottom of the shoulder capsule ligaments. As this progresses through the years, if you don't fix the kyphosis, the bottom part of the ball of the shoulder joint will continue to bump into the bottom of the socket. This will cause new bone spurs down there, which will further limit motion. In addition, the rotator cuff muscles will also begin to fail from all of that extra stretching. Finally, this new shoulder position will predispose you to more impingement (where the rotator cuff and biceps tendon get pinched).

So, what can you do? First, in the early phases of this kyphosis, you can beat it by using constant stretching against the grain of the forward head and shoulder movement. Here are some of my personal favorites:

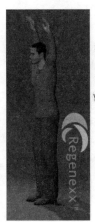

Lift your arms above your head and pinch your shoulder blades, feeling the stretch in your chest. Now lift and lengthen your body while bending very slightly back. You should feel it all the way down in your abdominals.

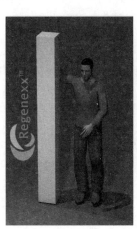

Find a door frame to stabilize your forearm and elbow. Gently push your body forward while you straighten your spine, feeling the stretch in the chest. Remember to do both sides.

In the later phases (once the spine bones have changed shape), you'll likely need professional help. In any case, if these stretches into extension cause significant neck, upper back, or lower back pain, you may have already had bone changes. Another possibility is that the facet joints in your spine may be arthritic or painful. Either way, you'll need to see a physician, like one of those in the Regenexx Network, if this is happening.

Roll up a towel or use a foam roller and lie back and stretch the front of the chest. You can vary your arm positions up and down. You may want to have the towel or foam roller extend to your head and neck for better support.

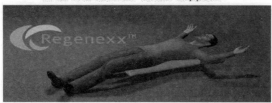

Are there regenerative injection treatments? If the shoulder ligaments on the bottom of the joint are lax, injections to tighten these ligaments (like the inferior glenohumeral ligament [IGHL]) can be very helpful. In addition, if the main shoulder joint has arthritis, stem cell injections into the joint may help. The same holds true for degenerative tears in the rotator cuff, which, based on our treatment registry data, respond very well to precise stem cell injections.

The Fight against Gravity! More Things to Do at Home

We all know that aging is a fight against gravity. Yet with stem cells in the mix, we can understand it differently. For example, as discussed in this chapter, that forward head and hump some people get in their upper back is merely gravity plus bad posture plus stem cells. What I mean by that is that any position of a joint or a part of the body held long enough will cause the local stem cells in bone to react, changing the shape of the bone.

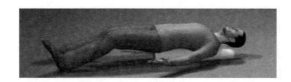

What are some simple things to do to fight this change in bone shape? Work against it! Above is an example of using a foam roller to fight the kyphosis (head forward position) that I explained earlier. For this exercise, the <u>foam roller (the white cylinder above) is easily purchased as an inexpensive fitness item</u>. A rolled up towel also works well. When you first begin, lie like this to get a sense of if it hurts. If it causes pain, then stop and see a doctor. If it doesn't, then start with 5 minutes once a day and work up to <u>more-advanced exercises</u> and longer time periods (15 minutes). Any part of your body that's beginning to change can be dealt with in the same way.

Is Your Belly Frying Your Facet Joints?

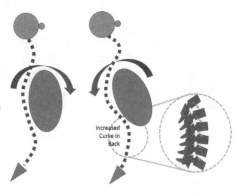

Your back hurts, and like many Americans you have a belly. Could there be a connection? We discussed how changes in the curve of the spine can cause either the discs or the facet joints to get overloaded. If you look at the image to the left, note that a big belly will want to topple you forward. There's just no way to stay upright without compensating. How does that work? You'll have to naturally increase the curve in the low back to move the center of gravity of the belly backward. In doing so, as the blowup in the diagram to the left shows, your body weight gets transferred from being evenly distributed between the discs in the front of the spine and the facet joints in the back to being more on those joints (the red arrows). Over time, this will cause your facet joints to get arthritis.

Scoliosis: A Side-Bent Spine

Your spine should be perfectly straight when viewed from the front. However, the spine can also bend to the side in a disease called scoliosis, especially in tall women. This can cause the shoulders and pelvis to become unbalanced. To the right, see how much havoc this can cause in the body, as the pelvis where the hips connect is way off.

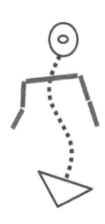

Also, it shouldn't be a surprise that when your shoulders are off, like the ones to the right, the forces on the ball and socket joint there will be very different.

What about when the side curves are more subtle? This is where many of us live, slight curves in the neck or back.

What Did I Self-diagnose in the Symmetry Screen?

So far, we've been discussing the concept of poor stability caused by too much movement, or hypermobility. Equally important is hypomobility, or where a joint or spinal segment doesn't move enough in all directions or certain directions. This is what you self-diagnosed in the five-minute symmetry screen.

Chiropractors and osteopaths have been focusing on hypomobility for more than a century. The reason we medical doctors have given them a hard time is that hypomobility has been traditionally hard to measure. However, there is good evidence now that this does occur. In fact, studies that specifically apply this concept (hypermobility versus hypomobility) show that patients with spinal hypermobility treated with exercise do better than patients with hypomobility. This makes sense because if you have too much mobility, you need to get the muscular stability system back online with exercise or other treatments to restore muscle function. However, patients with hypomobility did poorly with stability exercise. Why? They need more mobility, not more stability. This group did better with manipulation to force these segments to move.

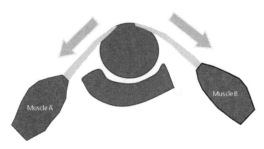

Hypomobility can be as damaging as hypermobility. The take-home message is that if your joints don't move normally in all directions, you have to get them to move normally or this will place more wear and tear onthe certain parts of the joint. What are some examples? If your knee won't straighten all the way, the front of the joint cartilage will wear more than the back. How about a hip that won't turn out all the way? The inner part of the hip will wear more than the outer.

Take, for example, this simple model of a joint and the muscles that help control that joint's movement. We have a ball-and-socket type joint with a ball sitting in a shallow socket (like the shoulder). Here we'll call them muscle A and muscle B. Both muscle A and B pull equally on the joint. When one pulls harder, the opposite muscle lengthens equally to allow the joint to move.

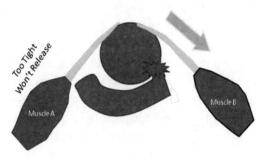

So as this joint moves, the ball stays in the middle of the socket. In fact, keeping the joint aligned with millimeter precision as it moves is critical. What happens if one muscle can't release as the other pulls? Now the joint moves too much to one side, banging into the side of the socket. This is an example of muscular hypomobility, where trigger points in one muscle make it tight and weak (more on this topic at this link). How do you fix this problem? You need to loosen up the tight muscle. This is discussed further in the neuromuscular section. The same thing can happen if one part of the joint capsule (the thick fibrous covering of the joint that helps to limit motion) is too tight or the ligaments that hold the joint together are too tight.

Adhesive Capsulitis: What Happens When the Joint Locks Down?

While it's clear, above, that a joint that doesn't move freely may have issues with overloading certain parts, what happens when the joint loses almost all of its motion? This is what happens in adhesive capsulitis. Nobody is 100% sure why this happens. Some think it's due to chronic inflammation in the joint due to poor blood sugar control,

This problem is most common in the shoulder and lesser recognized in the hip. In the shoulder, it tends to get noticed quickly, as the patient has to get any motion there from the shoulder blade against the chest wall rather than the shoulder joint. In the hip, it just tends to go hand in hand with arthritis, but often goes unnoticed. In the shoulder and hip, the loss of range of motion severely overloads small sections of the joint, which only tends to make arthritis happen faster.

We've had great success in both joints treating this range of motion problem using what we call pecutaneous capsuloplasty. This involves injecting platelet growth factors into the joint (the same ones we use in an epidural) and overdistending the capsule to break up the scarring and adhesions. This tends to free the joint and allow motion while hopefully leaving healing growth factors around to help things repair. In the hip, this is critical, as our treatment registry data there shows that outcomes with hip stem cell procedures are poorer with less range of motion of the joint.

Realignment Surgery: If I'm Asymmetrical, Won't Surgery Help?

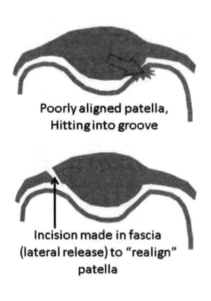

Poorly aligned patella, Hitting into groove

Incision made in fascia (lateral release) to "realign" patella

When I was in residency, one of my most- and least-favorite rotations was through pediatric rehabilitation. While it was always fun to be around the kids, these particular kids all had severe physical deformities. The surgeons on this rotation were great heroes, often allowing these kids to walk or function better by adding an inch here, taking away an inch there, or cutting this or that tendon. These kids were so severely disabled that it simply didn't matter that the accuracy of the surgical healing could be off by a few millimeters either way.

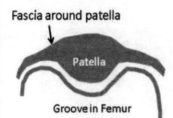

Fascia around patella

Patella

Groove in Femur

Fast forward 20 years, and I no longer see disabled kids for a living but patients with chronic joint and spine pain. I have seen hundreds of patients through the years who have undergone the same type of realignment surgeries, although they didn't do so well. What's the difference? The normal musculoskeletal system is tuned to submillimeter to millimeter precision. Human accuracy and surgical healing can be off a few millimeters either way. So, while it's possible that a surgically realigned tendon, muscle, ligament, or bone might be in the perfect anatomical position, it's more likely that it will heal "a little off." Also, many times these surgeries ignore the cause of the problem. Take the example of a <u>knee lateral release</u>. The concept is that the patella isn't tracking properly and is being pulled too far to the outside of its groove (or doesn't have enough pull toward the inside). Rather than asking what biomechanical forces have caused this to occur (issues in the hip, low back, etc.), we often try to take a quick fix approach by cutting some of the <u>quadriceps</u> attachment and <u>fascia</u> on the outside. Since the patella is aligned to submillimeter precision, and the surgery can only have accurate healing to a few millimeters, I often see that the patella is misaligned after the surgery. For example, if the lateral side scars and heals too tight, the patella will be too far lateral, or if too much of the lateral side is cut, too far medial. Add in to that calculus that the same forces that were pulling the patella too far laterally are likely still there (say too little hip external rotation), and the surgery hasn't solved the cause. Since these are permanent realignments of the musculoskeletal system, rather than a quick decision, I tell patients to think long and hard before getting a procedure that can't easily be undone.

Learning More About How the Parts Fit Together: Nonsurgical Solutions

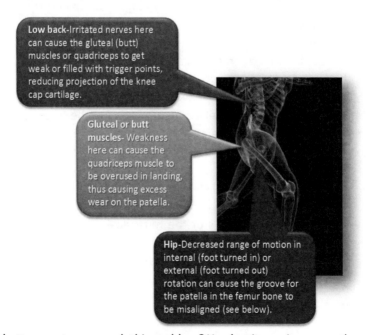

Misalignment due to patella moving to one side or femur groove turning: Problems in the big quadriceps muscle can cause the patella to move too much to the inside or outside, increasing wear. At the same time, rotation of the femur groove (from the hip or foot) can cause the same thing to happen.

Femur Groove

So, we just learned that trying to fix small alignment errors that can lead to big problems over time with surgery isn't such a good idea. Is there a

Low back-Irritated nerves here can cause the gluteal (butt) muscles or quadriceps to get weak or filled with trigger points, reducing projection of the knee cap cartilage.

Gluteal or butt muscles- Weakness here can cause the quadriceps muscle to be overused in landing, thus causing excess wear on the patella.

Hip-Decreased range of motion in internal (foot turned in) or external (foot turned out) rotation can cause the groove for the patella in the femur bone to be misaligned (see below).

better way to approach this problem? Yes, but it requires more thought. You know the song: "The hip bone's connected to the leg bone..." The same applies here.

We'll start by breaking down the patellofemoral problem above. The kneecap sits in a groove and is controlled by the surrounding structures (see below). There are two ways the kneecap can rub against the side of the groove. The first is that the kneecap moves out of position and bangs against the side walls of the groove (straight arrows). The second is if the groove itself moves (curved arrows). The groove sits in the femur bone and that bone's motion isn't controlled at the knee but at the hip. So, to fully understand kneecap problems, we must first start with the hip and work down. The femur bone, where the kneecap groove lives (trochlear groove), can move out of place if the hip doesn't have normal motion. The hip range of motion can be controlled by many things, not the least of which is arthritis at the hip. Irritated nerves in the low back can also lead to muscle firing issues in the hip or thigh muscles, which can also impact both the way the hip and kneecap move. Finally, weak muscles due to trigger points can also cause abnormal hip motion. In summary, what happens at your hip impacts your kneecap. Now let's look at the knee area. The kneecap is a just a small bone that lives at the end of one of the most powerful muscles in the human body: the quadriceps (aka "the quad"). What happens to these four muscles that make up the quadriceps determines what happens to the kneecap. I'm always dumbfounded when patients show up and are more concerned about the cartilage loss under their kneecap than the status of the main muscle that controls it. The problem is that outside of a short stint in physical therapy, nobody has ever told them that they should be concerned about the muscle. What can happen to the quad? Trigger points in the muscle can lead to parts of it being shut down, so this means that one part of the muscle pulls more than the other on the kneecap. Obviously, trauma to the kneecap can knock off cartilage, leading to arthritis. Finally, weakness in one of the muscles that make up the quadriceps (the VMO, or vastus medialis oblique) can also cause more outside pulling on the kneecap than inside pulling, leading to alignment problems.

Finally, we have to look below the kneecap to see if anything in the foot and ankle can also lead to problems. The angle of how the foot strikes the ground can impact how the femur groove is rotated at the hip. This will impact the knee as well.

In summary, looking at a kneecap problem as only being caused by this bone is a bad idea. It's also related to what happens in the low back, hip, and foot and ankle. So, if you see a physician for a kneecap problem, and he or she only focuses on the knee, other possible causes of your problem are being ignored. Why wouldn't all physicians look at the problem this way? Many times, its lack of training, but sometimes it's because our medical care system rewards more for procedures on a join than it does for diagnosing how the joing got that way.

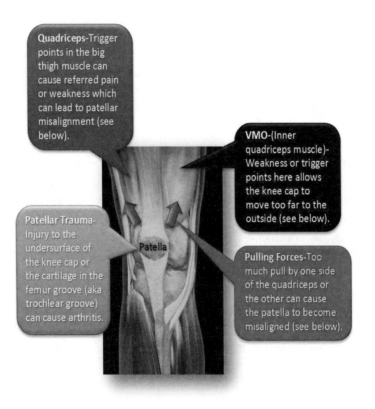

Quadriceps-Trigger points in the big thigh muscle can cause referred pain or weakness which can lead to patellar misalignment (see below).

VMO-(Inner quadriceps muscle)- Weakness or trigger points here allows the knee cap to move too far to the outside (see below).

Patellar Trauma- Injury to the undersurface of the knee cap or the cartilage in the femur groove (aka trochlear groove) can cause arthritis.

Patella

Pulling Forces-Too much pull by one side of the quadriceps or the other can cause the patella to become misaligned (see below).

More Specific Joint-Alignment Issues

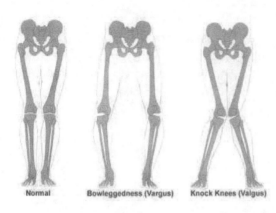

Normal   Bowleggedness (Vargus)   Knock Knees (Valgus)

Now that we've learned about the complex alignment of something as simple as a kneecap, let's look at some more obvious ones. First, the knee can be side bent just like the spine can. You've likely heard the term knock-kneed or bowlegged. These are conditions where the knees can be bent so that they touch (knock-kneed, or what doctors call valgus) or are too far apart (bowlegged, or what doctors call varus).

While people can be born this way, the leading cause of one knee going side bent is the removal of all or part of one meniscus surgically, which causes that one side to lose its spacer. The knee then collapses toward that side, putting much more pressure on the cartilage, which can lead to more arthritis. One solution often proposed is a high tibial osteotomy (HTO). This is a surgery where a wedge of bone is removed from the lower bone of the knee on the high side to even out the forces. <u>The good news is that it does seem to help</u>. The bad news is that it's a big surgery, and one way to prevent ever having to do this is to not remove pieces of the meniscus in the first place.

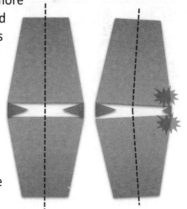

Foot Pronation

Foot pronation causes too much compression of the outside knee compartment

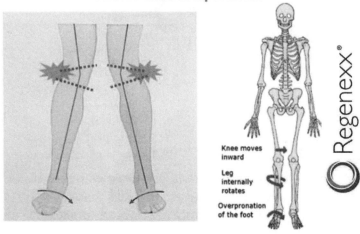

When your foot rolls inward, this is called pronation. This can cause knee and hip alignment issues, such as knock-knees. This can also cause the hip to internally rotate, overloading different parts of both of those joints. So sometimes, correcting a knee issue means correcting what's going on at the foot. Pronation can also be caused by irritated nerves in the back making the supporting leg muscles weaker.

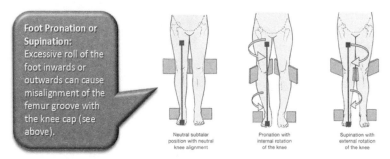

Foot Pronation or Supination: Excessive roll of the foot inwards or outwards can cause misalignment of the femur groove with the knee cap (see above).

The Master Control System for Body Symmetry

The upper neck is a special area with respect to alignment and posture. We've all heard about the balance system that involves the inner ear. However, our balance system is very complex. A bit like a

NASA spaceship, it has triple redundant systems, so that if one fails to provide enough information about balance, another system will automatically take over. This makes sense, since the loss of balance perception is not compatible with leading an active life and fending for yourself. Our balance system, therefore, has three inputs (as shown on the right): the inner ear, the eyes, and the upper neck joints. For many years, the focus has only been on the inner ear, but these other two systems are equally important and play into symmetry.

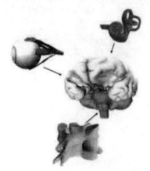

What part of the upper neck seems to be the most important for body symmetry? A number of years ago, a team of researchers started killing the little nerves that took information from the C2-C3 joints. The goal was to help alleviate the pain associated with these joints. While the pain got better, these patients all became very dizzy. The researchers were confused. While they knew about the inner ear being involved in balance, they didn't know about the upper neck. This misconception still exists in medicine today, with the vast majority of doctors not knowing about "cervicogenic dizziness," or dizziness coming from the neck, despite published research on the phenomenon. Based on the research, the C2-C3 area and upper neck muscles, as well as the sternocleidomastoid muscles, all seem to be implicated.

So, what does this have to do with alignment? Recently, some Australian researchers have determined that patients with whiplash injuries have difficulty in determining which end is up. Literally, their necks don't have the same proprioceptive ability as normal subjects. We believe that this is due to injury of the upper neck joints, which is common in this type of injury. We also see this same type of problem in patients who have injured the upper neck in the past or, for some reason, have chronic arthritis at C2- C3 or the high upper neck.

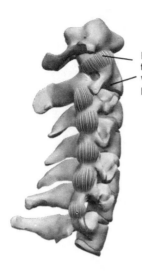

Injury to the joints of the neck can cause vertigo and visual problems.

These patients often have a head tilt. When I correct the head tilt on exam so their heads are straight, they feel crooked. Why? The upper neck joints are giving bad information about normal posture. This bad data causes the patient to tilt the head, but this strange position feels normal to the patient. The "<u>righting reflex</u>" then kicks in to keep the eyes and head level while standing. This causes the patient to tilt the body to one side to compensate, as the neck stays bent. This then causes all sorts of problems with arms frequently getting numb (usually on the little-finger side of the hand) from <u>thoracic outlet syndrome</u> (the nerves in the shoulder getting pinched). In addition, notice above how this causes the spine to bend sideways and can impact areas all the way down to the pelvis. It can even alter how one side of the leg and foot strikes the ground. As a result, in looking at alignment, one must always consider how it interfaces with this master balance-control system.

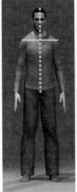
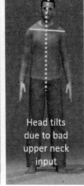
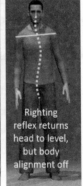

Head tilts due to bad upper neck input

Righting reflex returns head to level, but body alignment off

Can Alignment Be Impacted When the Spinal Stability System Goes Off-Line?

You've already learned about the stability system in the low back (<u>multifidus muscle</u>). Is there something similar in the neck, and can it impact alignment? We asked ourselves that question about 10 years ago. One of our physical therapists was tasked with seeing if the multifidus muscle in the neck showed signs of atrophy, like in the lower back. He was able to prove (later as part of his PhD thesis) that this does occur. When these small segmental stabilizers go off-line, something else has to kick in to stabilize the neck. In the neck and shoulder, the muscles that kick in are the trapezius, levator scapula, and scalenes (and sometimes jaw muscles). These muscles were never designed to be stability muscles, so they quickly get overloaded. As they get tighter to stabilize the neck, they can bring one shoulder higher. This causes the attachments of the muscles to get angry, as they were never designed to handle this type of excessive loading. This is called enthesopathy and is discussed

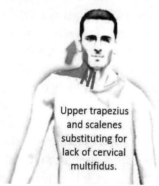

Upper trapezius and scalenes substituting for lack of cervical multifidus.

elsewhere. In addition, the upper trapezius and scalenes both have nerves nearby or traveling through them, so when they get too chronically tight, these nerves get in on the act. For the upper trapezius, the occipital nerve can get irritated, causing headaches. For the scalenes, the brachial plexus can get pinched, again leading to thoracic outlet symptoms with numbness in the little finger of the hand (ulnar or lower trunk of the brachial plexus distribution).

The Great Adaptation Machine

Our bodies were designed to keep moving at all costs and are great at adapting to problems that may develop in the human machinery. In a preindustrial society, the amount of physical prowess it took to collect, hunt, process, and consume food was great. In such a society, the potential for injury from a runaway animal or even a rockslide was also great. The only way for us to be able to get injured and keep going was to design the musculoskeletal system to be an adaptation machine. What does this mean? At its simplest, let's take a left-foot injury. With an injured left foot, you instinctively limp on the left and transfer more weight to the right. This takes weight off the left so it can heal. This strategy works, because we were meant to heal on the run. For example, <u>studies where patients are asked to bear more weight on an injured or operated area (different from the current nonweight-bearing orthopedic healing paradigm) show that healing with weight bearing is better than extended periods without weight on the joint.</u>

The great adaptation machine also gets a good deal more complex. I have noticed that in chronically injured patients, the system is constantly rearranging forces to be able to off-load certain areas. An example is my own minor chronic neck, upper-back, low-back, and leg symptoms. At times, my left scapula will hurt; at other times, my biceps tendon; and at others, my low back. I can feel my body rerouting forces through adaptation, from one site to the next. When the neck stabilizers go off-line, or when they are too taxed from my heavy weight-lifting routine, the big neck muscles take over, and the upper trapezius, levator scapula, scalenes, and SCM fire up. What happens when these muscles complain too much? My body reroutes the forces to the front of the shoulder by moving the scapula forward, but this aggravates the biceps tendon. If this causes the biceps too much pain, my body reroutes those forces by turning the rib cage, which causes the low back to get torqued, and so on. This complex neuromuscular response has allowed us for millennia to continue to function with injury.

For patients and medical practitioners, this adaptation process can often be like peeling back layers of an onion. Again, at its simplest (the injured left foot analogy), since the left foot is causing a limp, it may come as no surprise to the patient that the right foot begins to hurt as a result of excessive use. However, most patients fail to recognize the more complex adaptations. This means that they are completely unaware that the problems in all of these areas are related. In addition, physicians will often only go for the "low hanging fruit" of where it hurts today. This approach again avoids the salient question, how did all of this get this way? In addition, just treating the part that hurts will only be a temporary fix, as this part will soon be overloaded again!

How Do I Know if I Have an Alignment Problem?

First, I've only scratched the surface here concerning common problems with alignment. The goal was to introduce the concept, not list all things that an experienced musculoskeletal expert would see in daily practice.

At its simplest, patients with alignment problems have one-sided pain or arthritis in the absence of specific trauma. For example, while they may have both knees that hurt, the right hurts much worse than the left. In addition, an MRI or X-ray of both knees shows one has much more severe arthritis than the other. Examples of alignment issues can often be seen when looking in a mirror or asking your friends. You may notice that one shoulder is higher than the other, or the head is slightly tilted to the right or left, or that one hip is higher. Looking at wear patterns on clothing and shoes can give more clues. For example, does one shoe wear more than the other? Does one part of the sole of one shoe wear more than the other parts? Does one part of your pants wear out faster than another? Is it easier to hold a handbag or backpack on one shoulder or the other? When you're active, are you dramatically stronger on one side versus the other (more than you would expect based on being right or left handed)?

If I Have an Alignment Problem, What Else Can I Do About It?

The good news is that there are many therapists and practitioners who specialize in alignment. These concepts really began shortly after the turn of the century, when traditional allopathic medicine was in its infancy and unable to address what seemed like obvious problems to nonphysicians. The pioneers were Moshe Feldenkrais, Ida Rolf, and Matthias Alexander. I was introduced to these geniuses when I realized that by the early 1990s (just out of residency) these issues were still not being addressed by physicians. The concepts I've discussed here were not part of my training in physical medicine and rehabilitation. To remedy this deficit, I took to reading the old works of these masters to try and learn what I had never been taught as a physician. Newer systems such as Pilates, Muscle Activation Technique, Myofascial Release Approach, and Egoscue have added to the diversity of treatment methodologies that address various aspects of posture and alignment. In addition, <u>curve restoration</u> has now become a scientifically vetted medical art.

A caution, while some physical therapists have spent years learning advanced biomechanics, they are few and far between. The standard course of physical therapy education contains very little about how to identify and address common alignment problems. This is despite one of the early geniuses of muscle function actually being a physical therapist (<u>Florence Kendall</u>). So, if you've tried and failed physical therapy, it's unlikely that you saw a physical therapist with proper training in the art of biomechanical and alignment analysis and treatment.

Brief descriptions of the alignment concepts follow. Click on the links to learn more.

- <u>Rolfing</u>: Sounds a bit like the vernacular for vomiting, but it's actually named after the founder of the method, Ida Rolf. The focus is on very rigorous deep-massage techniques to free up areas of muscle and fascial tightness with the goal being to restore normal posture and alignment. This is generally accomplished in 10 sessions.

- <u>Alexander</u>: Matthias Alexander was a turn of the century orator in a time before the electric amplification of voice. He figured out that certain head and neck positions allowed the speaker to project his or her voice better in an auditorium. This was later applied to "sick" performers to improve their performances. This is now a system of treatment focused on head and neck alignment popular with stage and theater performers.

- <u>Muscle Activation Technique</u>: Developed by athletic trainer Greg Roskoph and based on the concept that certain muscles can become less active based on injury and certain patterns of movement, the focus is on balancing the moving biomechanics of the body by "turning on" these inhibited muscles.

- <u>Myofascial Release</u>: Pioneered by Arizona massage therapist John Barnes, the focus is on trigger point massage to release or free up tight muscles leading to poor body alignment. There is less focus on overall body posture than in Rolfing.

• <u>Egoscue</u>: Begun by Pete Egoscue, this system focuses on activating and strengthening specific muscles with specific exercises to restore normal body alignment and posture. This system has become popular with physical therapists wanting to increase their knowledge about biomechanics.

• <u>Feldenkrais</u>: Developed by Israeli physicist Moshe Feldenkrais, the focus is on alignment in simple movements.

• <u>Curve Restoration</u>: The gurus of this now scientifically vetted field are the Harrisons, chiropractors who have been publishing their results in peer-reviewed medical journals for years. They use very specifically designed forms of specialized traction to restore the normal curvature. They have also designed home units so that patients can try to deal with this problem in a do-it-yourself program.

Chapter 5: Neuromuscular

STABILITY
The ability of a joint to tightly move as it was designed without extra motions that might hurt the joint.

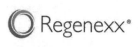

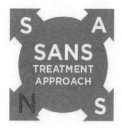

www.regenexx.com

ARTICULATION
The health of the joints. Shock-absorbing tissues like cartilage; spacer tissue such as meniscus; or stabilizing tissues such as labrum can be damaged.

NEUROMUSCULAR
The nerves drive the muscles. Nerves that are irritated or compressed cause pain and may be less able to promote muscles to properly fire.

SYMMETRY
The left/right and front/back balance of the body. When the body is asymmetrical, certain parts get injured or wear out faster.

"My countrymen should have nerves of steel, muscles of iron, and minds like thunderbolt."

Swami Vivekananda

Neuromuscular

For many readers, the term "neuromuscular" is a new term. To clarify, as it's used here, it means both nerves and muscles and is often used to refer to the <u>connection between the two</u>. While the nerves in various parts of the body tell many different organs what to do, the most visible organ they direct is muscle. Your nerve says, jump, and your muscle says, how high?

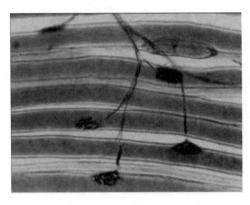

Think of the <u>nerves</u> as the wires that connect the main computer (the brain) with the <u>muscles</u>. You think of a movement, and the brain generates a nerve impulse that drives muscles. Information also goes the other way, from the skin, muscles, joints, ligaments, and tendons up to the brain. This information is called "<u>proprioceptive</u>" and allows you to finely adjust your movements to what's going on in your environment. For example, if you step on something unstable, you might fall. However, that information is quickly relayed to the spinal cord where reflex patterns stored there instantly adjust your stance.

It's easy to see how the nervous system plays a big role in the type of muscular spinal stability discussed in the first chapter. As discussed above, this type of stability during movement is made possible by <u>proprioception</u>, which is used to provide real-time feedback so that a moving joint stays in finely tuned alignment. For example, if the joint experiences forces that might cause it to translate or shift too much, small joint sensors detect this motion and instantly tighten muscles to counteract that abnormal motion and keep the two joint surfaces aligned (keep the joint in the neutral zone). If this didn't happen thousands of times each day, the joint would wear out much more quickly.

What happens when this system of sensors, nerve impulses, and finely tuned muscle firing goes off-line? As discussed earlier in the "Stability" chapter, all heck breaks loose. In this chapter you'll learn that when spinal nerve irritation or compression occurs, the muscular stability system for the spine goes off-line, and the spine becomes unstable. I believe the same happens in peripheral joints, like the knee. If spinal nerves are irritated in the back (note: you may not feel any back pain), the muscles that help stabilize the knee in movement can go off-line or have reduced efficiency, and, as a result, the knee joint becomes unstable. So now, when the knee experiences abnormal forces, like a shift, the wiring loop through the spine between the joint sensors and the muscles that protect the spine is impacted, causing an ever-so-slight delay. This delay leads to a joint that gets out of alignment more easily during motion and, as a result, a joint that is more likely to become arthritic. Since this concept of muscular activation delay has already been very well documented for spinal stability (here the delay causes the vertebrae to become unstable in movement), there is no reason to believe it only applies to the spine.

One of the problems we've had as a medical community is our main and most widely available test for diagnosing nerve pathology (electromyogram [EMG]/nerve conduction study [NCS]) is very specific for certain types of nerve injuries (such as when a nerve is wholly or partially destroyed by trauma) but not very sensitive for other types of nerve problems. In particular, many significant problems with the nerves involve small fibers (small-fiber neuropathy); whereas, the EMG/NCS test can't detect this type of pathology. In addition, the test has very poor sensitivity in detecting nerve irritation. While other more sensitive nerve tests (in particular, quantitative somatosensory tests [QST]) are commonly used in research, they are not yet widely used by physicians. So, in a real way, physicians are often "flying blind" from a diagnostic-testing standpoint in figuring out when nerves are sick. In other words, based on the research, a negative EMG/NCS doesn't rule out nerve trouble. It's a test that's highly specific, but with poor sensitivity. The definition of a good diagnostic test is one which is highly specific and highly sensitive (capable of detecting the disease 99% of the time when it's present, and shows negative 99% of the time when the disease isn't there).

So, in summary, even small amounts of spinal nerve irritation may not cause any noticeable back or neck pain, but it can wreak havoc with the muscular stability system either in the spine itself or in your joints. Since this system protects your joints during activity, when this type of nerve problem takes muscles off-line or reduces their efficiency, this will eventually lead to less protection for the joints and an earlier onset of arthritis. In addition, the diagnostic-test toolbox we have available to us today doesn't include tests that are capable of detecting this type of nerve problem, hence, the reason this problem often goes undiagnosed. In addition, I believe that treating this problem is a key component of long-term joint preservation.

Take This Simple 10-Item Test for Nerve Problems

1.　　I have numbness, tingling, burning, or electrical sensations. Yes / No

2.　　I have chronic tightness that feels like pressure in my arm or leg with certain activities. Yes / No

3.　　I have a chronically tight muscle that just won't "let go" no matter how hard I stretch. Yes / No

4.　　I have pain in my wrist area whenever I reach for something. Yes / No

5.　　I have pain in the back or bottom of my heel that won't go away. Yes / No

6.　　One arm or leg always seems to be significantly weaker　or smaller than the other, no matter how hard I try to strengthen it. Yes/No

7.　　My arm or leg feels a bit "goofy" or uncoordinated after I do certain things. Yes/No

8.　　I have an area of chronic pain that just won't go away no matter what I try. Yes/No

9.　　I have chronic neck or back pain. Yes/No

10.　　I had a back or neck problem years ago, but it seems to be fine now. Yes/No

If you answered yes to any of the above, you may have a nerve/muscle problem and not know it. *Question 1* about numbness is more obvious. Most people associate these symptoms with nerve problems. *Question 2* isn't so obvious. When there's pressure on a nerve in the neck or back, many patients don't necessarily feel neck or back pain, but instead feel pressure in the muscle that is supplied by that nerve. Some patients describe it as feeling like a blood-pressure cuff is pressing on the muscle. *Question 3* is also not obvious. That chronic hamstrings or groin tightness you've been blaming on being out of shape could actually be caused by a pinched or irritated nerve. *Question 4* is really interesting. We commonly see this when there's scarring around the median and/or ulnar nerve. Reaching out to get something places the nerve on stretch, and since it's scarred, it can't move with the arm, which causes pain where the nerve is scarred down. How about *question 5*, the heel pain? Most patients with plantar fasciitis would think it must be caused by something in the arch of their foot. However, we see patients every day who have S1 nerve problems in their back or a pinched tibial nerve at the ankle who have this problem caused by an irritated nerve.

Question 6 may seem more like something associated with a nerve, but the weakness or atrophy (smaller muscles) I'm talking about is where one arm or leg is notably smaller, not the kind you see in paralysis. *Question 7* is an extension of 6 as sometimes patients with nerve problems note that their arm or leg seems uncoordinated. *Questions 8 and 9* are connected, in that a bad nerve can cause pain just as readily as it can cause numbness, tingling, or burning. Finally, it's important to note in *question 10* that many patients who no longer believe they have any back or neck problems because the pain has gone away still have bad nerves that cause problems in joints, muscles, and other areas.

Arthritis Doesn't Cause Pain; Pain Causes Arthritis

I saw this title come across a science news feed a few years back. It hit me like a welcome pie in the face as I had often suspected that something like this had been happening in my patients. The concept is simple, yet it will change the face of orthopedics and rheumatology forever. What was discovered? That irritated nerves can cause bad chemicals to dump into joints, which leads to cartilage breakdown. Since that time, many other articles have been published confirming this link between bad nerves and bad joints (see here, here, and here). This discovery is equivalent to when we doctors learned that stomach ulcers were caused by bacteria and not stress (I was taught in medical school that ulcers were due to stress). How can arthritis be caused by pain? The authors created an elegant animal model that showed that nerve activation in a joint leads to bad chemicals being dumped into the joint, which leads to pain and faster onset of joint arthritis. This is a reverse of what has traditionally been considered (i.e., that a joint is injured and begins to degrade and then causes pain). It's important to stop for a moment to consider how these scientists have turned orthopedics on its head. Again, our entire orthopedic care model is based on the concept that injury in a joint (or accumulated injuries over a long period of time) leads to arthritis in the joint, which leads to more joint breakdown and pain. This new model reverses the old paradigm so that now it's aggravated nerves that lead to arthritis. Sound familiar? I believe this is just an extension of what we've been discussing here: problems with spinal nerve irritation lead to bad chemicals being dumped into a joint and a "sloppy" joint with poor stability, which ultimately leads to arthritis.

I have had my own knee problems caused by my back. Using this new model, my knee problems were caused by spinal nerve irritation (which I never perceived as low-back pain) causing not only a sloppy knee joint (due to parts of the big stabilizer muscles being shut down by trigger points) but also bad catabolic (breakdown) chemicals dumping into the joint. This issue was quickly fixed not by operating on my knee or even injecting magic stem cells into the knee, but by bringing the spinal and joint stability systems back online by using IMS to get rid of the trigger points. What are trigger points? Read on.

Low-Level Arthritis Pain vs. Nerve Pain

Based upon my clinical experience and this new model of nerve-related joint pain and arthritis, I would place patients into two distinct categories: what I'll call "neuropathic arthritis" versus "classic arthritis." Early on in the degenerative process, and for some patients who have more of a spinal component to their joint pain, patients are firmly in the "neuropathic arthritis" (NA) camp. These patients have severe joint pain that is often disabling or can become disabling with certain types of activity. I see these patients in the clinic, often very desperate because their joint pain is very intrusive. They are either completely disabled by 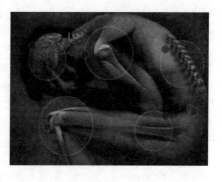 their pain or they are unable to exercise at high levels. In this new model of joint pain, these patients have an active spinal nerve problem manifesting as joint pain. They are often unaware that this joint pain is linked to their spine, but if you dig enough, they will usually admit to a history of spinal problems that have either (in their mind) been successfully treated (perhaps with a surgery many years in the past) or are ongoing, but the pain is low level and (in their mind) under good control. They have usually had several unsuccessful joint surgeries, which didn't work because while they have issues in the joint, they also have active issues in the spine that were unaddressed by their joint surgeries. Treating the spine in these patients can often make a huge difference.

The second camp is the traditional "classic arthritis" (CA). The CA group no longer has an active spinal component, or if they do, their arthritic joint has long since degenerated. Their pain pattern is different and matches what we know of arthritis pain. You may remember your grandparents being stiff in the morning with low-level pain that became better with activity as the joint "warmed up." Just like gramps and granny, once these patients start moving, they generally feel better. Treating the spine in this group is often too little too late, as the joint damage is done.

It's important to note that there are other factors at play in many of these patients, so this is a simplified discussion. For example, patients with joints that are unstable from a ligament standpoint may also have more pain when they are active, and patients with bad joints due to severe trauma may have less pain as their joint warms up. Like anything in medicine, the body is a very complex machine, hence, the

SANS approach, which looks at all components of the musculoskeletal system.

So, What Can Be Done to Fix the Spinal Nerve-Joint Connection?

Despite research showing that irritated spinal nerves may be associated with joint problems, most physicians have a hard time associating joint pain with a low-back nerve problem. The first step in identifying a spinal nerve component as a cause of joint pain is simply a thorough neurologic exam. When I say a complete exam, I don't mean the "Can you feel this?" type of neurologic exam. This careful exam is focused on comparing sensation from side to side and on the same side, testing multiple different types of sensation. This includes not only light touch (the *can you feel this* exam) but also pain sensation (pinprick) and perhaps hot/cold sensation. The exam also recognizes that there are multiple types of pain and nerve referral patterns, including those from spinal joints, nerve trauma, and muscle trigger points.

If the exam shows that spinal nerve irritation may be occurring, the next step is a spine MRI. Correlations between the exam findings and the MRI are important. In addition, this correlation acknowledges that while spinal nerves can be compressed by bone spurs and herniated or bulged spinal discs, they can also be irritated by sloppy stability in the spine (see the "Stability" chapter). An MRI marker of this type of sloppy stability can be seen on MRI as multifidus muscle atrophy (see the "Stability" chapter). So even though there may be no bulging disc on the spinal nerve, significant atrophy of the deep stabilizers at this level (multifidus) combined with sensation problems at the nerve in the leg means that the spinal segment is likely sloppy from a muscular-stability standpoint.

Treatment for Irritated Spinal Nerves

Your spine has discs, which act as shock absorbers. The diagram to the left shows that the spinal discs can herniate their inner contents (nucleus pulposus), which can place pressure on spinal nerves. This is called radiculopathy (if more severe) or radiculitis (if less severe). This has also been called "sciatica," although this is not an accurate term.

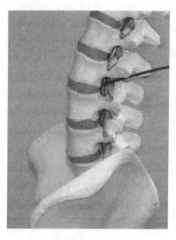

The traditional solution is to surgically remove the herniated portion of the disc sitting on the spinal nerve. In the 1940s, this was a great advance. Patients with numb and weak legs due to a bad back now had a treatment. On the other hand, it began our current move toward invasive spine treatment, a path that many have criticized.

Treatment for herniated discs remained largely surgical until studies in the 1980s showed that a few years after the disc herniation, results for patients treated with surgery weren't all that different from those who didn't get surgery. What emerged from this research was the revolutionary idea that perhaps herniated-disc patients could be treated without surgery.

As a result, the focus began to shift toward conservative management, which by the late 1990s included epidural injections. This meant placing strong anti-inflammatory medications around the painful and swollen spinal nerves. At first these injections were just adapted from pregnancy epidurals, which are usually provided to control the pain of labor, but later these evolved to more specific placement of medication between the disc and swollen nerve. These newer injections were called transforaminal injections (literally meaning through the foramen, or into the hole in the spine where the spine nerve exits). Transforaminal epidural injections of anti-inflammatory seem to work better than the older pregnancy epidural injection types (interlaminar and caudal).

The conventional wisdom regarding epidural injections is that we wait until the patient has failed a significant course of medications, physical therapy, and time. While this makes some sense from a cost-savings standpoint, our newer understanding that irritated spinal nerves can lead to shrunken spinal-stabilizing muscles and instability means that earlier intervention is likely warranted. I believe that preservation of these spinal stabilizers is very important and that the goal of treatment is to bring them back online early by calming down swollen and irritated spinal nerves. My own example is important. Several years ago, I was performing heavy dead lifts from the floor early in the morning (generally a bad idea). I felt a pop and went down on the ground. My pain was so severe that I couldn't walk, stand, move, and so forth. Had I stayed like this for any length of time, my spinal stabilizers would have quickly atrophied, leading to months of rehab to get back into shape. Instead, I had my partner perform an immediate epidural to calm these swollen nerves and was back to weight lifting three days later! This is what I mean by "early intervention."

The Paradigm Changes Again: Epidural Steroids are Toxic

You may have seen that steroid epidurals have been all over the news of late. First, there was a compounding pharmacy contamination tragedy that led to many sick patients because the steroids being injected weren't sterile. Next came the revelations that the steroids used in these shots caused women to lose bone mass at an alarming rate (worsening osteoporosis). Other studies have shown that the steroids can also shut down important brain responses that help you deal effectively with stress. The conclusion? Injecting these high-dose steroids into the back or neck can cause significant side effects, but it generally works.

Is there another way to get the same or a better result that avoids steroids? Rather than big dose anti-inflammatories, we believe that the next generation treatments will be using much lower dose medications and combining these with regenerative medicine. So rather than injecting 80 mg of corticosteroid (the height of the Empire State Building), injecting smaller physiologic doses of steroids and adding in level II (or even level III) regenerative medicine solution.

To do this, we have pioneered using the growth factors from the patient's own blood platelets (platelet lysate) instead of these toxic steroids. So rather than using a sledgehammer to treat the swelling (steroids), we use growth factors that can reduce swelling and improve blood flow. Does it work? We tracked 232 patients in a registry and compared patients getting

Traditional steroid epidurals (85 people) and platelet lysate (Regenexx-PL- Disc procedure—147 patients). The function questionnaires (functional rating index [FRI]—a higher score is better) showed more improvement in the platelet epidural patients than the steroid epidural patients (see graph on next page).

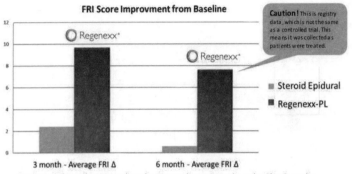

Details: n=60 for patients responding after PL procedure at 3 months and n=48 at 6 months.
N=24 at 3 months for steroid epidural patients and n=19 at 6 months.

Can We Use a Platelet Lysate Injection to Fix Damaged Nerves?

In medical school, I was taught that while a damaged nerve might be able to regenerate a little bit over time, most nerve injures were permanent.

Recently, one of our physicians, Ron Hanson, MD, investigated whether nerves might be helped by injecting the nerve. The simplest form of this procedure is called nerve hydrodissection. Basically, fluid is injected around the nerve using very strict ultrasound-imaging injection protocols. This frees the nerve up from any scarring that may cause pain. Next, platelet lysate is injected to help the nerve heal. We've seen some very interesting results in select patients with everything from severe chronic nerve pain (complex regional pain syndrome [CRPS]) to more specific nerve damage. We remain cautiously optimistic and will continue to move forward trying to help these patients who have few good options.

Making the Transition from the Nerve to the Muscle

You've learned about the nerves. Now you have to learn about where the nerves go—the muscle. We like to think of these as separate structures, yet one look at the former Superman actor Christopher Reeve in his wheelchair shows they are not. A spinal cord injury in his neck shut off all nerve input to the muscles. What happened? He went from being one generation's Superman to being shriveled up. Why? The nerve and the muscle are one continuous structure. What happens to your nerves directly and immediately impacts the muscles.

The Nerve-Muscle Hotspot: Trigger Points

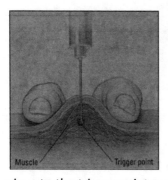

Muscle   Trigger point

Trigger point injections (TPIs) were first popularized by Janet Travell, MD, one of JFK's physicians. Janet's techniques made it into popular medical culture because JFK had a bad back that often responded well to her trigger point injections with numbing medicine. Sometime later, Canadian neurologist Chan Gunn, MD added a significant piece to the trigger point puzzle. Travell had noted that just using a needle without injecting anesthetic (dry needling) seemed to work just as well. To the medical establishment of the day, this seemed like voodoo. At the time, Chinese acupuncture was largely unknown in the West, so Travell largely placed her emphasis on injecting anesthetic and anti-inflammatory medications. Gunn grew up in Korea, where a more aggressive form of Korean muscle acupuncture was common, so he moved forward with Travell's dry needling technique, substituting the much finer and less traumatic acupuncture needles for the more traumatic cutting - edge injection needles used by Travell. Gunn also

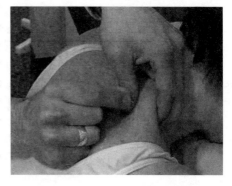

theorized that the muscle trigger points that Travell thought were due to overuse were more likely caused by nerve irritation. The science of the last 20 years supports Gunn's theory that nerve problems (autonomic and likely spinal nerve) and trigger points are closely related. By the early 1990s, while physicians who were experts at trigger point injections were few and far between, TPIs were used by a plurality of doctors treating musculoskeletal pain. Then something happened that often drives the course of medical care much more than efficacy or science—the reimbursement changed. Prior to the mid-1990s, a physician could receive adequate compensation per site injected. After the mid-1990s, the average compensation for this procedure was reduced by about 70%–90%! In addition, getting compensated by insurers became more difficult. This was all it took to relegate the art of trigger point injections to the history books. Today, because of this reimbursement collapse, finding a physician experienced in managing this type of muscle pain is like finding a needle in a haystack (pardon the pun).

I think my own personal story is important. In the late-1990s I attended a medical conference that involved days of sitting. For an unknown reason, my left knee began to ache and swell. There was no trauma to the knee. I was literally hobbling around the office, and all my aerobic exercise came to a screeching halt. I underwent an MRI, convinced that I had somehow torn a meniscus or some cartilage. While the MRI showed the swelling and perhaps some questionable small tears in the meniscus it didn't show a "smoking gun" cause for my severe pain. I went to see an orthopedic surgeon who wanted to perform a diagnostic arthroscopy, likely chop out some meniscus and remove a "plica." I was desperate and convinced the MRI was missing the true cause, so I reluctantly signed on for surgery. A few days before the planned surgery, a visiting doctor from Canada was in our clinic and asked if I had tried trigger point therapy in my quadriceps muscle and low back? I said no, looking at him like he was some alien speaking in tongues. At this point, I had seen the best physical therapists in town and failed all of their exercises, so I was desperate. I told my Canadian colleague that I would try anything. Turns out, this visiting physician was one of those "needles in a haystack" as he was experienced in the Gunn trigger point

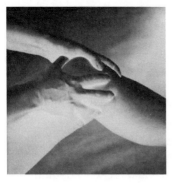technique (called IMS, short for intramuscular stimulation). He examined my thigh muscle (quadriceps) and my low back, pulled out an acupuncture needle, and proceeded to stick this in my low back and thigh muscles. The muscles cramped suddenly as the needles hit the trigger points (more strange than painful). After a two minute treatment, I got off the table and walked normally. That night, I went running for the first time in months, without a twinge. I canceled my surgery and have never looked back. I was so impressed, I learned the technique and began using it in patients.

IMS has revolutionized our practice, providing relief to patients who would only otherwise be treated by much more invasive treatments. Because of reimbursement issues (insurers don't generally cover IMS, and the other form of trigger point therapy [TPI] is poorly reimbursed), the technique has remained obscure. There may be other reasons the technique has never moved to a wider physician audience, as it takes significant effort and dedication to learn how best to apply the procedure to get consistent results.

At a medical conference where both traditional Chinese acupuncture and IMS were being taught, I had insight into how my medical colleagues view this complexity. After Dr. Gunn lectured about IMS, I turned to the physician sitting to the left of me and asked, "Wow, isn't this IMS stuff great?" Her response was, "It's too complex. You have to learn where all the muscles are, what they do, where to put the needle for each one, what to avoid...with traditional Chinese acupuncture, I just look at a chart on the wall and put the needle at X marks the spot." So while traditional Chinese acupuncture (placing a needle into the skin at specific Chinese chi points) has become popular, IMS has remained in obscurity.

These past few years, IMS has finally taken a leap forward by being adopted by various Colorado physical therapists (PT). One of our former PTs who we had trained in IMS went through the red tape to

<u>allow physical therapists to widely practice the technique after very intense coursework</u>. As a result, IMS is now gaining more acceptance, and more patients are getting more access to the technique through physical therapists.

What if I Don't Have Back Pain?

Let me again use my own example. While I no longer had back pain when my knee went out, how did my low back cause a knee problem? How does that work?

On that fateful day at the end of the medical conference, muscle trigger points in my spine and thigh caused severe knee pain and swelling. Did I have a back issue? Turns out, I had fractured a few little bones in my back about 10 years before the day I had my knee pain. Other than a few bouts of mild stiffness, I had never had any ongoing back pain after the fractures, just a sudden and unexplained onset of knee pain. So, what's the connection? The upper low-back spinal nerves were irritated, which caused big trigger points to develop in my quadriceps thigh muscle. As this happened, large sections of that big muscle began to shut down, turning off the major stability system of the knee, which began to swell because of the extra wear and tear due to abnormal motion. Why didn't my back hurt? Pressing on spinal nerves generally doesn't give you back pain, it causes symptoms where the nerve innervates (the area the nerve supplies). So, if I took magic fingers and pressed on the right-L5 spinal nerve in your back, you would feel it in your right leg and big toe, not your back.

Enthesopathy

We take for granted that our muscles not only contract but also have a function as shock absorbers, letting go in a controlled fashion. As an example, when you jump from a fence at a height of just four feet, your femur bone should break. Why doesn't it? The big quadriceps muscle absorbs the shock by acting as an <u>eccentric contraction</u> (controlled release). When a muscle has trigger points, the biomechanical properties of that muscle change. Large sections of the muscle can lose their ability to act as active shock absorbers. We believe this leads to extra pull on the areas where the muscles attach to the bone. This causes swelling and breakdown of these areas known as <u>enthesopathy</u>.

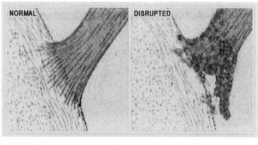

Enthesopathy means that where a tendon attaches to bone, the tendon is aggravated and swollen. If this goes on a long time, you may see small tears in the ligament. If it gets really severe, you may see bigger tears. All of this can cause pain.

While many physicians will recognize problems in joints, and fewer will recognize trigger points in muscles, in our experience, even fewer will recognize enthesopathy. This is a problem, as many patients suffer from this problem. The good news is, a new generation of physicians armed with PRP to treat tendons and ultrasound imaging to detect problems in those tendons is finally beginning to address this important problem.

What Are Common Areas of Enthesopathy?

Head: The back of the head where the trapezius, sternocleidomastoid, and suboccipital muscles insert is frequently an area of muscle-attachment overload. These muscles can irritate the greater and lesser occipital nerves, leading to headache.

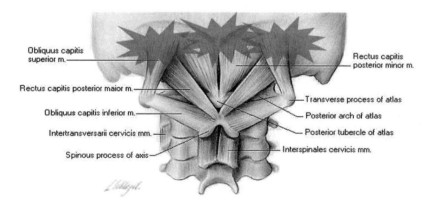

Elbow: The classic medial and lateral epicondylitis (golfer's and tennis

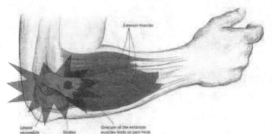

elbow) are attachment sites for muscles that get overloaded. We see this commonly in patients who have nerve irritation in the neck or shoulder (cervical radiculopathy or radiculitis and thoracic outlet syndrome).

Upper Back: The back of the ribs where the iliocostalis and quadratus lumborum muscles insert can become inflamed and lead to back pain. We see this commonly when the multifidus stabilizers are off-line.

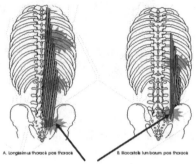

A. Longissimus thoracis pas thoracis   B. Iliocostalis lumborum pas thoracis

Tennis Elbow of Low Back

Lower Back and Pelvis: The posterior superior iliac spine (PSIS) area is where many large low-back muscles take their anchor. As already described, we consider this the tennis elbow area of the low back. Patients can often point to a single spot just to the side of the upper tailbone (dimples of Venus). This spot gets overloaded as the stabilizer muscles go off-line. Ischium ("Sit Bone"): This is an area where the hamstrings muscle attaches, as well as many other important deep pelvic muscles. Patients with enthesopathy here have trouble sitting or have deep buttocks pain. This is more common in patients with a

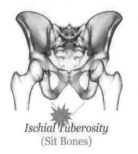

Ischial Tuberosity
(Sit Bones)

lower lumbar nerve irritation and/ or problem with sacroiliac (SI joint) instability.

Posterior/Lateral Hip Girdle: This is one of the most common areas of tenderness in women (and many men) who have problems in the SI joint or with lower spine nerves. These powerful buttock muscles attach to the bone here and travel south to the back and side of the hip.

Greater Trochanter: The side of the hip is where many important muscles attach.

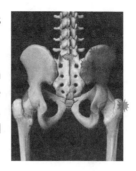

Knee—Pes Anserine: This area is a common insertion for many muscles that travel in the front of the thigh, including the sartorius, gracilis, and

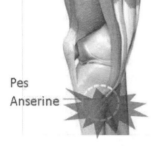

Pes Anserine

semitendinosus. These patients have pain on the inside of the knee that is below the joint and is often confused with meniscus tears. We see this problem in patients who have low-back issues leading to knee pain.

Knee—Hamstrings: The hamstrings are muscles that make up the back of the leg and attach to the back of the knee. They're responsible for helping to set the position of the bottom knee bone on the top thigh bone and for helping the knee meniscus position itself correctly. They can become painful at the back inside or outside of the knee. This pain is often confused with a torn meniscus. We frequently see this happen when the S1 nerve in the low back is fired up. Patients may not recognize that a back problem is causing the pain at the back of the knee as all they may feel is that their hamstrings are chronically tight.

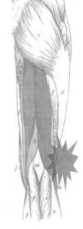

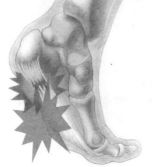

Foot—Plantar Fascia: At the bottom of the foot near the heel is a strong fascia that extends from this area to the base of the toes called the plantar fascia. This area helps to support the arch and acts as a shock absorber for the foot. Where this tough fibrous structure originates in the heel can develop enthesopathy. In particular, we see this happen quite a bit when patients have an S1 nerve problem in their low backs.

What Happens When Tendons Have Bigger Problems?

We've discussed what happens when tendons attached to bone are overloaded and aggravated. What happens when they fail? For partial tears, in our experience, platelet rich plasma (Regenexx-SCP) works well. For complete tears, where the pieces haven't retracted back like rubber bands, same-day stem cells tend to work well. For full-thickness retracted tears, where the ends have snapped back, surgery is likely needed (although we're working on nonsurgical options). Tendons can get partial or complete tears like ligaments. Here is a list of the most common ones we see:

Shoulder—Biceps Tendon: The biceps muscle is the big one you see in the front of the arm. It attaches through its tendon to the top of the main shoulder joint and becomes one with the lip around the shoulder socket (labrum). It can be irritated and cause pain in the front of the

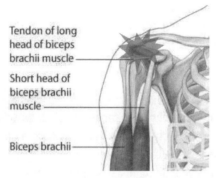

Tendon of long head of biceps brachii muscle

Short head of biceps brachii muscle

Biceps brachii

shoulder or get torn (usually where it originates at the shoulder labrum), which is called a SLAP tear. The tendon can also have partial or degenerative tears inside it, often caused by rubbing on the other shoulder structures due to poor biomechanics. Sometimes, surgeons will try to cut the ligaments on top of this area (called a shoulder decompression), but this can leave the shoulder more unstable.

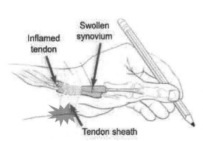

Inflamed tendon

Swollen synovium

Tendon sheath

Thumb—Blackberry Thumb, Texting Thumb, Gamer's Thumb, De Quervain's Tenosynovitis: The tendons on the back and outside of the thumb can become swollen or degenerated. In our experience, this is frequently associated with carpal tunnel syndrome and problems with irritated nerves in the neck. The latter can cause the thumb muscles to misfire and irritate the tendons.

Iliopsoas: This muscle starts in the low back and travels frontward toward the inside of the hip. It's responsible for helping to lift the leg. The tendon can become irritated or get partially torn if the front of the hip is overloaded, for example from too much curve in the low back. It can also be injured in kicking sports. The tendon can also snap over the hip. A common cause is problems with upper low-back nerves that provide nerve supply to these muscles.

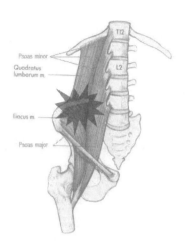

Hamstrings: The hamstrings muscles at the back of the leg start at your buttocks area and travel downward. They actually originate from the ischial tuberosity (the bone where you sit). This is an area where they can become torn or just irritated. This can cause pain in the buttocks area as well as pain or tightness in the back of the leg. The lower lumbar nerves in the back can also cause problems in this muscle and tendon.

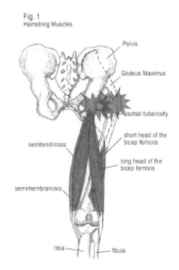

Fig. 1
Hamstring Muscles

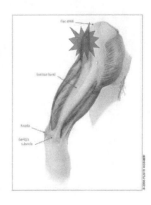

Iliotibial Band (ITB): This is an area at the side of the hip and leg that begins from the top of your hip and extends down to the knee. Patients with chronic instability in the sacroiliac joint tend have problems here. The ligament is rarely torn, but can be irritated.

Achilles Tendon: This is the thick tendon at the back of your ankle and heel. It connects your calf muscle to your heel, so it's responsible for pushing you off as you walk. It can get torn in middle-aged and active-elderly patients, usually during sports performed beyond current fitness level. It can have partial tears inside the tendon or can tear completely by snapping back like a rubber band. It's also very common in patients who have S1 nerve problems in the low back.

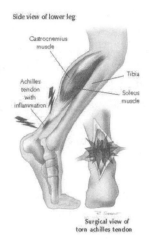

Side view of lower leg

Surgical view of torn achilles tendon

Peroneal Tendons: These tendons on the outside of the foot and ankle are involved in stabilizing the foot when you're balancing on one

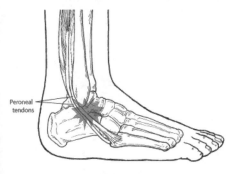

leg or when you're on one leg while walking or running. They can become torn (commonly they can split down the middle). Usually this isn't from a specific injury, but from wear and tear. This problem can be associated with instability in the ankle ligaments as the tendons try to stabilize the foot and ankle, something they weren't designed to do. They can also become torn when there is a chronic lower lumbar nerve problem leading to abnormal firing of the peroneal muscles.

Extensor Hallucis Longus (EHL): **This is the tendon that raises your big toe. In patients with chronic foot and ankle issues, it can become misaligned so that it no longer travels across the main toe joint but is displaced more toward the inside. It can also become raised and overloaded and sore/painful, especially when walking or hiking. This tendon is commonly impacted** when the nerves in the low back are chronically irritated, and as a result, the position of the foot andankle changes. <u>See this link for further discussion and diagrams</u>.

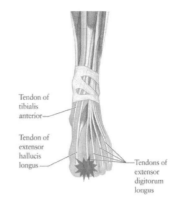

An Example of Healing Tendons: The Regenexx Rotator Cuff (RC) Procedure

As I've stressed, rotator cuff surgery is dicey business. Many patients don't heal as expected because the tendon failed due to problems with blood supply, degeneration, and lack of stem cells. Hence, sewing an unhealthy tendon back together doesn't work well. How can you get the tendon healthier? In our experience, we've seen great results when the patient'sown platelets or stem cells are injected with precision guidance into the torn rotator cuff tendon. Click on the video below to see more details:

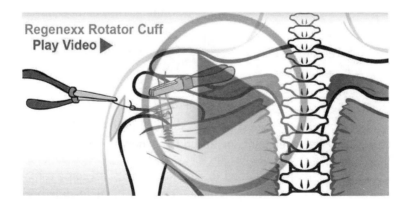

Regenexx Rotator Cuff
Play Video ▶

How Instability and Enthesopathy Are Often Linked

You've learned about instability, now let's learn about how an unstable joint often leads to "pissed off" muscle attachments. Basically, in this case we have muscles that are pulling too hard on their bony attachments. How does this work?

Have you ever tried to stand up in a row boat? The "ground" you're standing on is unstable, as it seems to randomly move in unexpected ways. The amount of energy it takes to do anything, even reaching for an oar, is tremendous. The same happens when a joint is unstable. In the case of your body, when a joint is unstable the muscles automatically kick into overdrive to compensate and stabilize the joint. When your muscles do this for long periods of time, the places where they attach to bones can get irritated.

For example, this commonly occurs when the spinal stability system goes off-line. Look at the picture of the spine and note just some of the many spine muscles that act between spine bones (from one vertebra to the next). Imagine if all of these were working overtime because the spine bones were unstable due to a bad ligament. The places where these muscles attach would be on fire, as these attachments would be overloaded (enthesopathy). This is why many spine-injection approaches often 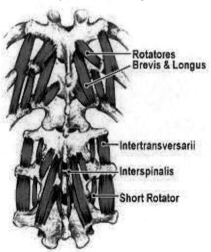 fail, as medical practitioners fail to inject these areas in favor of nerves and joints. For example, we can inject medications into a specific structure, like the facet joint, or around the nerves, but if these tendons attached to these small segmental muscles have been damaged due to years of overuse, then placing medication in a joint or around a nerve (which are different locations than these muscle attachments) won't help the pain. We also frequently see this around the SI joint and hip girdle (see Case 1: SI Joint Shirley).

Multifidus Atrophy

In the first chapter, you were introduced to spinal instability. This often happens because the muscles that stabilize the spine become weak. How does this happen?

If you have numbness, tingling, or weakness in an arm or a leg, you meet the classical definition of spinal nerve root compression called radiculopathy or radiculitis (literally in English, root disease and root swelling). Getting to a diagnosis in this instance is usually routine, as long as there is something on your exam that correlates with a pinched nerve on your MRI (bone spurs or a disc pressing on a spinal nerve). However, if you have more subtle signs of nerve-root irritation or nothing structural on your MRI, you're less likely to get a diagnosis.

You also learned in the first chapter that your MRI may be harboring "secrets" (or at least important information that the radiologist neglected to read). If you look at your MRI, you may be able to see this problem yourself. This finding is easy to see if you think of the spinal muscles as a steak. A steak in the grocery store is a cross section of the muscles, just like the axial view of an MRI. If you find the axial view of the spine and open those images, in the low back (where this finding is commonly seen), it will look like the image to the left. The multifidus muscles will be in the back of the spine (to the bottom of an MRI image). This area looks like a steak.

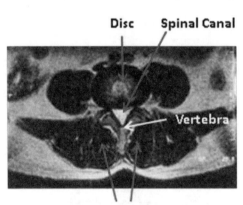

Disc   Spinal Canal

Vertebra

Multifidus

More Details on How to Read Your Own MRI Images for Multifidus Atrophy

Open your MRI CD. You will see different "sequences." These are different parameters for how the MRI was taken. There may be five to seven different ones listed. First, choose the axial T2 sequences (these might be labeled AX T2, Axial or Ax STIR, or AX T2 FSE). If you don't see "T2, " just pick the axial or ax sequence that looks like the image below, with a whitish circle in the middle (the fluid in the spinal canal) and lots of white to the left and right of the spine (your love handles). These images usually start at the top of the sequence (upper part of your low back), so take a look at the dark areas in the back of the spine (the middle to bottom of the image behind the white circle). This area looks very much like a steak you would buy at the grocery store (see image on right). Why does it look that way? Because a steak is a cross section through muscle, and so is this picture.

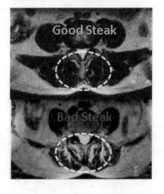

Now scroll down through the spine, paying attention to the steak part. Look for what I call "the bad steak," or where the muscles look fatty (see the image below—you want to look in the white-dashed area for whitish coloring in the otherwise dark muscles). As you start to get to areas where multifidus atrophy shows up, you'll likely be toward the bottom of the spine (higher image numbers in this sequence). To help guide you, the illustrations on the next page are from one of the original research papers that first described this problem (authored by Kader et al.). Note that the area in the white dashed circle has a bit of white (fat atrophy) in the mild picture, more white in the moderate, and is 50%-or-more white in the severe. We routinely see patients in our office with 80%–90% white in this area by the time they see us. Again, look at all levels on the axial images for these white areas.

Why is this important again? Multifidus atrophy has been associated with both chronic low-back pain and leg pain. Why? The muscle acts as a stabilizer of the vertebra (as discussed in the first chapter). If it gets weaker and smaller, it can't stabilize as well, and this can lead to nerves getting irritated.

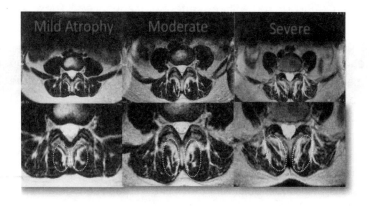

Mild Atrophy   Moderate   Severe

The Tennis Elbow Spot of the Low Back

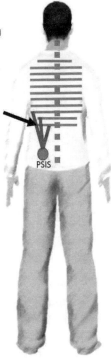

Long back extensor muscles like the quadratus lumborum and iliocostalis lumborum that attach to the ribs, start substituting for the mutifidus being off-line. This causes the spot where they originate (PSIS-here the blue circle area) to become chronically swollen.

PSIS

After many years of examining patients, I can tell you there's always one spot that's tender in about 60% of all low-back-pain patients: the posterior superior iliac spine (PSIS). Why? When stability problems manifest in the low back, we tend to see the big muscles that attach the pelvis to the ribs substitute for the smaller muscles. This includes the quadratus lumborum and iliocostalis lumborum, both of which originate at a common attachment point in the low back on the pelvic bone (see figure). This is a similar situation to the <u>lateral</u> and <u>medial</u> <u>epicondyles</u> of the elbow, where the muscles of the forearm attach and can cause <u>tennis elbow</u> or <u>golfer's elbow</u>. This common low-back attachment site is the <u>PSIS</u>. We consider this the tennis elbow site of the low back. This spot is the dimple (also called "<u>dimples of Venus</u>") just on either side of the upper tailbone. This type of chronic pain due to tendon pulling is called an <u>enthesopathy</u>, which is better explained in a later chapter.

Peripheral Nerve Entrapment

A "peripheral nerve" is simply one that instead of living in your spine, lives in your torso, hips, arms, legs, hand, feet, and so on. The nerves that course through your body sometimes have to make it through some tight spots. The more common tight spots have lent their names to common medical maladies, like "carpal tunnel syndrome" (the tight spot for the median nerve in your wrist). These common tight nerve areas are in all parts of your body.

Here is a list of common areas where nerves get entrapped and cause symptoms.

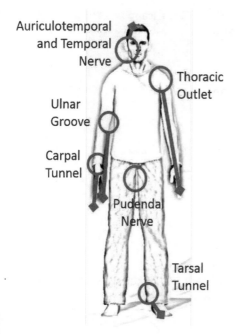

Auriculotemporal and Temporal Nerve

Thoracic Outlet

Ulnar Groove

Carpal Tunnel

Pudendal Nerve

Tarsal Tunnel

Auriculotemporal and Temporal Nerve: This is a common cause of headaches on the side of the head and temple area.

Thoracic Outlet: Impingement of a nerve in this part of the shoulder/rib complex causes numbness and tingling down the arm, often in the little finger.

Ulnar Groove: This area in the back inside of the elbow is your "funny bone," where the ulnar nerve goes through its groove. It can cause numbness in the little finger.

Carpal Tunnel: This common area of pressure on the median nerve can cause pain in the thumb or numbness or tingling/weakness in the hand.

Pudendal Nerve: This is a nerve in the groin that when entrapped can cause pain or numbness/tingling in the genitals or anus.

Piriformis Syndrome: This is entrapment of the big sciatic nerve as it travels through the piriformis muscle at the back of the hip. This can cause leg pain, numbness/tingling, or weakness.

Tarsal Tunnel: This is an area on the inside of the ankle that can put pressure on the tibial nerve as it travels to the foot, causing pain, numbness, or tingling in the heel or bottom of the foot.

Occipital Nerve: This is a nerve at the back of the head (there are two—greater and lesser) that is frequently compressed with loss of normal curve in the neck or with whiplash-type syndromes.

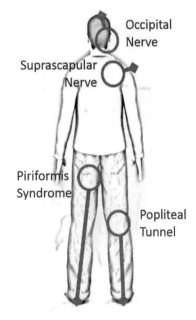

Suprascapular Nerve: This is an area at the back of the shoulder blade where an important shoulder nerve travels. Pressure on this nerve can lead to pain and weakness in the shoulder.

Popliteal Tunnel: This is an area at the back of the knee where the tibial nerve travels to the lower leg. It can become compressed when there is a Baker's cyst in the knee. The symptoms are leg and foot numbness, tingling, weakness, or pain.

Realize this is a short list of places where nerves can become entrapped throughout the body.

Superficial Nerve Syndromes

There are many places where nerves pass through small tunnels in the fascia that covers your muscles. These small tunnels are all over your body, and, recently, a physician from New Zealand (Dr. John Lyftogt) developed a technique to treat this type of pain. Basically, the area is localized on exam or with ultrasound (the small nerve appears swollen at one of these common tunnels) and injected with a solution to reduce nerve pain (usually 5% dextrose in anesthetic). This procedure seems to work well in chronic pain syndromes where the patient can localize certain areas on the skin or just below the skin that, when pressed, re-create the pain pattern. For example, a patient with pain on the outside of the knee where the skin nerve exits the kneecap fascia (the covering tissue of the outside of the kneecap). This area can be pressed on, and this reproduces the pain. Another

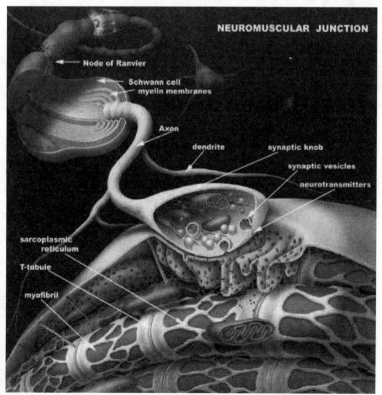

use of this technique can be in widespread pain where many injections are used at many nerve exit locations.

Really Bad Nerve Problems...
Problems at the Neuromuscular Junction: Painful Dystonia

The <u>neuromuscular junction</u> is where the nerve talks to the muscle. As you recall, the nerve talks to the muscle to tell it what to do. The nerve says, jump, and the muscle says, how high? Think of the neuromuscular junction as a room where one person is talking to another. The nerve does the talking, and the muscle listens. If the room is quiet, the instructions barked by the nerve to the muscle can be clearly understood. If the room is very noisy or the nerve isn't speaking clearly, the instructions may be misheard or misinterpreted by the muscle. The latter case is what happens in <u>cervical dystonia</u>. This is a nerve disease that when it's severe results in a patient with spasmodic torticollis, or where a patient has his or her head turned to one side on a permanent basis. However, like all diseases, this problem comes in less severe forms, where the patient just has constantly tight muscles that won't let go. This chronic tightness (called dystonia) naturally changes the alignment, which can lead to pain and other problems. I call this less severe form, painful dystonia. We see this in patients who have had traumatic nerve injuries (often in car crash trauma). In this case, the noise in the neuromuscular junction room is turned up, so that the nerve instructions to the muscle sound like "stay tight all the time," even when that signal makes no sense for the situation. This can be treated with medications like Myobloc that work to turn down the noise in the room so the muscle can hear the nerve instructions. Injected in enough quantity, this medication could turn off all signals from the nerve to the muscle, but injected in smaller quantities, it only reduces the noise in the room.

Central Sensitization

Let's say you're in your car and all of a sudden all of the warning lights start to go off. You take the car to the mechanic, and he or she says that there may be a few things wrong here and there with the car, but the real problem is that the wiring is bad. This is central sensitization

(CS) also known as complex regional pain syndrome type II, fibromyalgia, neural sensitization, and so on. In all of these conditions, it's an injury to the pain- reporting wiring of the body (the nerves and microprocessors that control them) that causes the problem. The nerves become hypersensitive to pain. This phenomenon has been extensively published—most references are for <u>whiplash</u> or <u>fibromyalgia</u>. <u>This problem is also now being discussed as related to joint pain (as discussed earlier)</u>.

Patients with CS simply have a nervous system that's on fire. At its early stages, it may cause arthritis (see above), but as this gets worse, large areas of the body can be impacted. In addition, these areas don't follow normal nerve pathways like dermatomes (skin areas associated with certain spinal nerves), so often times many physicians without training in this area label these patients as having "nonanatomic" sensation problems. These patients, as they progress, can't tolerate physical therapy, massage, injections, acupuncture, IMS, and so forth. <u>Our research group demonstrated that at an early</u> 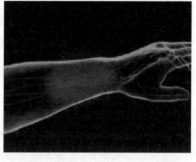 <u>stage, trigger points may make the sensitization problem worse</u>. At later stages or when more severe nerve injury has occurred, cold sensitivity is common. <u>For example, for patients with traumatic CS, a cold summer's night (about 60 degrees Fahrenheit) is actually painful as that's all it takes to activate pain nerves</u>. Think about this for a second: How cold would it have to be for a normal person, you, to perceive cold as pain? Below freezing? Twenty below? These patients feel this at less than 60 degrees.

CS patients are generally the most difficult patients to treat. First, the pain sensitivity levels have to be brought down to a more normal level. One way to do this is medication. We have seen many medications for this type of nerve related pain come and go— <u>Neurontin</u>, <u>Tegretol</u>, <u>Elavil (amitriptyline)</u>, <u>Doxepin</u>, just to name a few. They all had the problem in that they didn't work for most patients. However, newer nerve-pain drugs are just coming to market, with many new ones in the pipeline. The most effective drug we have seen is the newer drug <u>Lyrica</u>. This works well in about 6 in 10 of these patients to reduce nerve pain and "put some water on the fire." Once this is accomplished, the next step is usually to identify the problems that caused the fire. In many patients, there were specific musculoskeletal problems that led to others, which ultimately led to the fire getting out of control. Finding these specific problems and treating them can then start to provide relief. As an example, a patient labeled with "fibromyalgia" may note that his right neck and shoulder began hurting first, then his right low back, then his arm and leg. Tracing the issues back to the neck would be the way to approach this patient.

In addition, we are also encouraged with the results in using the nerve-hydrodissection technique with platelet lysate, as discussed earlier. This approach is to try and help the nerve function better by placing helpful platelet-derived growth factors near the nerve.

Neuromuscular Resources

Calming down nerves through injection often requires an expert trained in x-ray–guided procedures. Here are some resources:
- <u>ISIS (International Spinal Injection Society)</u>
- <u>ASIPP (American Society for Interventional Pain Practitioners)</u>

Realize that almost all of these physicians still use steroid epidurals as their primary injection type. **If you're interested in platelet lysate epidurals, see the** <u>Regenexx Network physicians at this link</u>.

The most effective way we've seen to address chronic trigger points is either through IMS or trigger point injections. Here are some lists of where to find these "needle in the haystack" doctors and physical therapists:

- <u>A list of Gunn IMS practitioners</u>
- <u>Trigger point educational group</u>
- <u>Physical therapists trained in IMS</u>

Trigger points in muscles can be difficult to treat on your own, but we've seen some success with these approaches:

- Electro Therapeutic Point Stimulation (ETPS)
- Thera Cane

Enthesopathy: See level 1 prolotherapy and level 2 PRP resources discussed in the "Articulation" chapter.

Getting Out of the Hole

The goal of the rest of this book is to provide additional information for those patients who want to go further in their understanding of their problems. To go from an educated participant in their own recovery to a leader of that recovery. I've only had a few patients make it this far in their understanding. One gentleman who comes to mind was an engineer from Canada who moved to Colorado to get care from our clinic. Over time, our office visits became more of me providing advice about his next steps and what might be wrong rather than the doctor leading the patient. At first it was a bit disorienting, but later it became fun.

If you're a patient who can't do much without things badly flaring up, this section is for you. First, you need read this whole book to understand what's wrong. Next, you'll likely need to make some hard choices and follow the process diligently. I call this "digging out of the hole."

What is "the hole"? Your body has all or most of these systems we've talked about seriously involved. Your stability is fried, your joints are beginning to or have already given out, your nerves and muscles are shut down and on fire, and your symmetry is all catawampus. It may take you one to two years to get all of this addressed and to "climb out of the hole."

Where Do You Start?

1.   **You must get "off the sauce."** We've seen an explosion in the prescription of narcotics by doctors after pharmaceutical companies claimed that newer long-acting and very addictive

narcotics weren't addictive. Narcotics also take away your natural ability to control pain. So, while they may take away the pain in the short run, they make the pain signals magnified in the long run. As a result, you must decrease and eventually eliminate your use of narcotics.

2.   **Reduce the pain** coming from various joints, tendons, muscles, and nerves. These problem areas must be first carefully identified. Often this will take an hour or more of hands-on exam, combining many different types of imaging, including ultrasound, MRI, and movement-based studies. Once the areas are identified, then the focus should be on precise biologic injections to ramp up the healing response in these areas.

3.   **Get rid of muscle trigger points** caused by irritated nerves using once or twice a week IMS. This will allow your muscles to begin to participate in providing stability.

4.   Slowly work on getting more stable and stronger. This may at first be at very low levels. For example, some patients may have to begin in the pool and then take a few months to graduate to simple and gentle land strengthening. It may take one to two years to work back up to anything resembling a big workout.

5.   Fix the bad symmetry that likely got you here in the first place.

The next chapter of patient cases speaks to a practical application of SANS and how some patients at various levels of disability made it "out of the hole."

Chapter 6: Putting It All Together

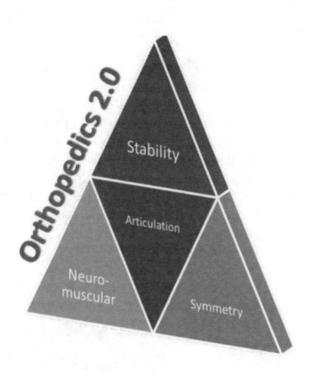

"The physician can bury his mistakes, but the architect can only advise his client to plant vines—so they should go as far as possible from home to build their first buildings."
Frank Lloyd Wright

My goal with this chapter is to present several patient examples, from less complex to more complex, so the reader can see how the puzzle pieces fit together and interact with each other.

Case 1: SI Joint Shirley

Shirley is a 54-year-old woman who fell and had chronic pain in the back of her hip. She had seen multiple physical therapists and chiropractors, obtaining only temporary relief. Patients, like Shirley, who complain of hip pain are often told they have pain coming from the hip joint. An X-ray is usually taken showing some arthritis, which would be common for her age. Based on little else than the report of hip pain and the X-ray, the patient is frequently scheduled for a hip replacement without ever confirming that it's her hip joint that is causing the pain. Isn't hip pain always from the hip joint?

To investigate the possible cause of hip pain, let's look at the pelvis. The picture to the right shows that the hip joint is

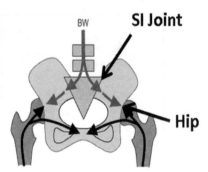

Trabecular system of the Pelvis
Follows Weight-Bearing Lines

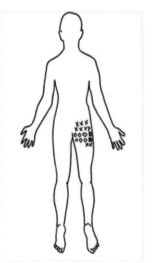

Common Pain Area
for SI Joint Pain

connected to the pelvis and that the next joint up the chain is called the SI Joint (short for sacroiliac joint). You can see that these joints are close together. Pain from either joint can cause patients to complain of "hip pain." The hip joint proper tends to cause more groin pain, and patients with SI joint problems tend to have more pain in the back of the hip near the PSIS area (see diagram to the left that shows a common location of SI joint pain). Truth is, either the hip or the SI joint can cause pain in the back or front of the hip, so how do we tell which is causing the complaint of hip pain? To determine the source of the pain, we performed diagnostic numbing injections. Under X-ray guidance (fluoroscopy), we injected numbing medicine into the SI joint and hip. Injecting the hip only minimally helped her pain, while injecting her SI joint took away 70% of her pain. We had our man!

Since we had injected ultra-low-dose anti-inflammatories in her joint, this gave her some relief for a few weeks, but the pain returned. Now the question was, what caused her to have chronic SI joint pain? Because of her fall on the SI joint area, we suspected instability, which was confirmed on exam (see SANS pyramid to the right). What other clues led us to believe that she might be unstable in the SI joint ? The patient had tenderness throughout the muscle attachments associated with the

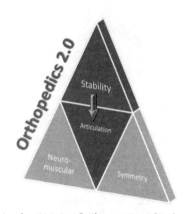

SI joint. The attachments of the gluteal muscles and piriformis showed signs of enthesopathy. At the back of the hip (greater trochanter), she was also tender where these muscles attached. If she had just injured the joint, this didn't make sense. However, if the joint was unstable, these muscles would be working overtime to

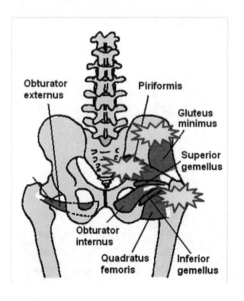

try and help stabilize the area, thus causing the enthesopathy. So, in addition to treating the SI joint, these other areas would need to be treated as well. Why? While they might go away if we fixed the stability issue in the SI joint, based on clinical experience, it was more likely that they would remain as the damage at these muscle tendon attachments had been done.

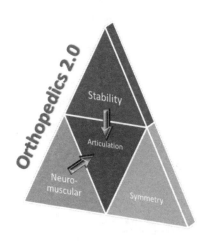

So what options are there to fix an unstable SI joint? Fusing the joint surgically with screws has been used, but fusion usually just transfers forces to the joints above and below, so we wouldn't consider this option. Most pain management physicians would either consider repeatedly injecting high-dose steroids into the joint or an SI joint radiofrequency procedure. As discussed in the "Articulation" chapter, high-dose steroids can damage the joint. Radiofrequency is where special needles or catheters are inserted to ablate the nerves that take pain from the joint. This is covered by many insurers, but these small nerves also provide proprioceptive input to the muscles that stabilize the joint, so nuking them could mean less active muscular stability. In addition, this would only address the joint pain and not the pain she was having from the enthesopathy muscle areas. In our experience, the only treatment that would be regenerative rather than ablative (build up rather than destroy), tighten the ligaments to help the passive instability, and address the areas

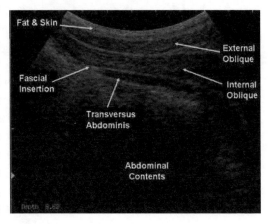

of muscle/tendon enthesopathy is prolotherapy. After two prolotherapy treatments, the pain was down by 75%. The next step was to address the likely muscular stability issues. <u>The muscular stability system for the SI joint is the transversus abdominus</u>. This is a tough muscle to teach patients to contract, <u>as it's the deepest stomach muscle</u>. However, we can easily see the muscle on <u>ultrasound imaging</u>, so we used this advanced imaging to help the patient have a sense of when she was contracting the muscle.

In summary, Shirley is a good case to understand how all the treatment choices and pieces fit together. Starting with identifying a pain generator and then asking why she still hurts (instability) and then looking at different joint treatment options and finally ending with a very specific rehabilitation component to address the muscular instability and weakness.

Case 2: Ankle Alice

This is a 55-year-old woman who was seen for an ankle problem that began after a climbing fall last year. She had multiple ankle ligament sprains as well as bone chips in the joint from trauma. After two surgical debridements, she wasn't much better. I have included below that show (on the far left) a normal ankle alignment between the tibia- talus-calcaneus bones (normal ankle MRI from someone

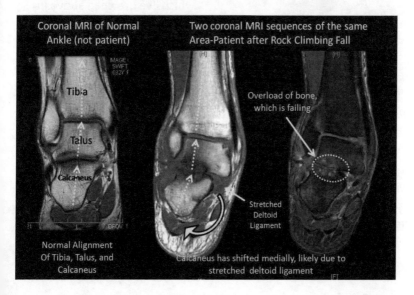

Coronal MRI of Normal Ankle (not patient)

Two coronal MRI sequences of the same Area-Patient after Rock Climbing Fall

Tibia

Talus

Calcaneus

Overload of bone, which is failing

Stretched Deltoid Ligament

Normal Alignment Of Tibia, Talus, and Calcaneus

Calcaneus has shifted medially, likely due to stretched deltoid ligament else-not the patient). With this type of normal alignment, when the patient steps down to walk, forces are generated that start at the bottom of the foot and move up through the ankle bones. I have drawn these forces here as the yellow dotted lines. Notice that these force lines are relatively straight in the normal patient MRI. The forces move from the calcaneus (heel bone) to the talus (ankle bone) to the tibia (lower leg bone). In this patent's MRIs in the middle and on the right (same coronal MRI slice—but different types of MRI sequences), you can see how the force line is shifted to the left. The calcaneus (heel bone) is rotated laterally (in these images—to the left), and as a result, there is overload of the bones and talocalcaneal joint (the yellow dashed line on the far-right picture showing light color in the otherwise dark bone). So, because the heel bone is now bent to the lateral side (left in the above pictures), the ground forces don't hit the talus bone evenly. Instead, the lateral talus and heel bone (calcaneus) are overloaded on this MRI, and the bone is so beat up, it's actually starting to die off (the dark color in the bone on the middle picture and the light color in the bone on the right picture).

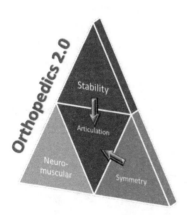

So how did the ankle get this way? Regrettably, nobody ever asked this question before. Her exam revealed a loose deltoid ligament, which I've drawn in above in the middle picture as a red-dashed line (" stretched deltoid ligament"). Think of this as living duct tape that normally doesn't allow the heel bone to move to the left (lateral). When this got stretched in her climbing fall, it all of a sudden allowed her heel bone to move laterally and redistributed the forces to the lateral side of that joint. This caused her cartilage on that side to wear out more quickly and the bone to be beat up. So, in order to fix this (we use injected mesenchymal stem cells; others might use different tools), you have to shore up the lateral subtalar joint (for us injecting her own stem cells into that joint) as well as tighten the deltoid ligament to try and prevent the overload from happening.

This example illustrates how Orthopedics 2.0 is about more than quick surgical fixes—it's about figuring out how the joint got to its current condition and then designing strategies using advanced tools (such as stem cells) to try and restore normal joint function. When we look at this versus the SANS pyramid, we see that the stability impacted both the joint (articulation) and the alignment.

Case 3: Unstable Mable

Mable is a 45-year-old white female who was in a rear-end car crash a few months prior to our evaluation. Immediately after the crash, she noted severe and sharp right-sided upper neck and head pain. When she is seen in the clinic, she's tender over the right C1–C3 facet joints, and her right upper trapezius, levator scapula, sternocleidomastoids, and scalenes are tight. She has headaches with pressure over the upper neck. What happened to Mable and why does she still hurt after several months?

The upper neck facet joints are commonly injured in rear-end car crashes. In addition, the upper neck ligaments can be injured as well. Mable gets good relief once we inject low-dose anti-inflammatories into the right C1–C3 facet joints, but that's only temporary. Her 3.0 ultra-high-field MRI shows that there is evidence of likely stretching of the ligaments that

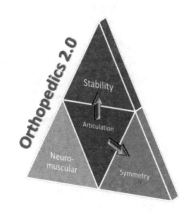

hold the head on (alar and transverse ligaments). I believe what happened to Mable is that once these structures were injured, the upper-neck stability muscles went off-line. There is good evidence in whiplash-injured patients that these muscles atrophy. What happens next? The big neck muscles take over. These are the upper trapezius, levator scapula, sternocleidomastoids (SCMs), and the scalenes. However, they weren't designed to be neck stabilizers, so their attachments get overloaded, leading to enthesopathy. This is what causes pain at the back of Mable's head and irritates the occipital nerves that exit near the attachment of the upper trapezius and SCMs. This leads to chronic headache (as well as the referred pain from the injured C1–C3 joints, which are known causes of headache as well). In addition, Mable was unable to bear weight on these injured joints, so her neck curve was lost as her body figured out how to offload the joints.

We injected the upper cervical facet joints where the high-field MRI of her upper neck showed problems in the ligaments that hold the head in place. The enthesopathy was treated by prolotherapy injections where the muscles attached to the back of the head. Once the facet joints and upper neck muscles were calmed down, Mable was able to strengthen her neck. She also underwent curve-restoration therapy to get back the normal lordosis. Once the joint pain, enthesopathy, muscular stability, and alignment were addressed, Mable dramatically improved.

Case 4: Sensitized Sally

Sally is a 40-year-old woman who was in a rear-end car crash who developed neck and back pain within weeks of the injury. At that point, she developed severe pain and numbness in her hands and feet as well as headaches. She was diagnosed with fibromyalgia and given pain medications.

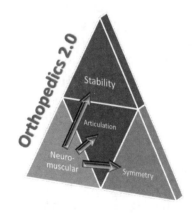

When she was first seen at our clinic, she had severe tenderness everywhere. She told me that attempts at physical therapy, massage, and trigger point injections had all caused days of severe pain. The patient was given a quantitative somatosensory test that demonstrated significant central sensitization. She was placed on Lyrica to help reduce her nerve sensitization. Once that began to reduce the severe pain, it became clear that multiple joints and muscles were being impacted by the nerve issues. Her posture had eroded, and the muscular stability in the low back was compromised.

Once the Lyrica began to help, we addressed the neuromuscular trigger points with IMS and the postural issues with Egoscue, and we injected multiple joints with low-dose anti-inflammatories to reduce pain. The patient also had an epidural in the low back to reduce nerve pain and rehabilitation to get the low-back stabilizers back online. The patient's pain then began to reduce. However, due to the nature of the nerve injury, she will require long-term pain management.

Case 5: Catawampus Wayne

Are you ready for a more complex biomechanical analysis? This one demonstrates how a little injury can eventually lead to bigger problems. This patient had a serious fall from a bike about three years ago. He injured his shoulder, kidney, and hip. When he was first evaluated for stem cell treatment of his hip, I was concerned about his low back.

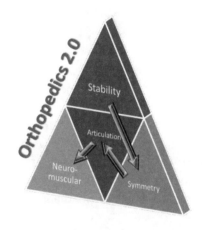

While stem cells in the hip helped the hip pain (he now walks faster through an airport), over the ensuing year, he continued to develop problems in his low back and leg. He was finally diagnosed with a cyst on his right L4–L5 facet joint that was pressing on a spinal nerve and giving him pain down the leg.

The facet joints are small joints in the back, and sometimes arthritis of the joints can result in a cyst (just like a swollen knee joint can develop a Baker's cyst). These cysts can press on spinal nerves, so they can be a double whammy for the patient. The patient had the facet cyst treated with a steroid injection to pop the cyst. This helped some of the leg symptoms and severe nerve pain, but by the time I reexamined him, his back was pretty bad (he was unable to stand straight). This was impacting his work as a physician. While knowing he had a facet cyst was a good start in helping him, asking the question of how he got that way was important if this was going to be successfully treated without surgical fusion of this level. His case is a good example of the Orthopedics 2.0 concept. Consider the Orthopedics 2.0 pyramid above in which I've filled in various portions. To better explain, more discussion and pictures are needed.

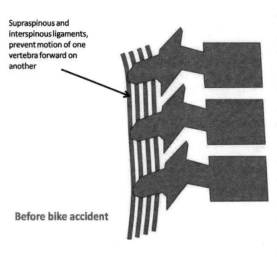

Supraspinous and interspinous ligaments, prevent motion of one vertebra forward on another

Before bike accident

On his flexion-extension views, it was noted that he had the L4 vertebra slipping forward on the L5 vertebra. This forward slippage was at the same level as his facet cyst. Coincidence? Likely not. The way to understand this problem involves some ligaments in the back of the spine that act as the major duct tape that help keep the spine aligned. These ligaments are the supraspinous and interspinous ligaments. The image to the left shows the ligaments (red lines) in the back of the spine.

So before his bike accident, these ligaments were doing their job, helping to hold the spine in alignment. The picture above shows that the ligaments are holding the vertebrae in

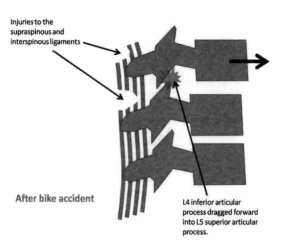

Injuries to the supraspinous and interspinous ligaments

After bike accident

L4 inferior articular process dragged forward into L5 superior articular process.

place. They act to make sure that all of the vertebrae stay aligned when you bend forward. They also control how much one vertebra is allowed to move relative to the vertebra above or below. Note that after the bike crash, the injury and tearing of these ligaments (gap in the red lines—see right) allow the L4 vertebra to move forward on the L5 vertebra. Since these ligaments help to hold the vertebrae in alignment when he bends forward, the facet joints move more than they can tolerate. This ultimately leads to excess wear and tear of these joints. Is there another part of this puzzle?

An interesting observation as he lies prone on the table is seen to the right. Why is there severe bulging of the left abdominal wall? Further questioning of the patient reveals that he also injured his kidney in the bike accident and had surgery on the left kidney. The scar can be seen in the picture to the right.

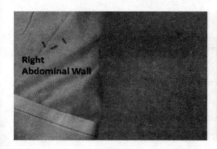

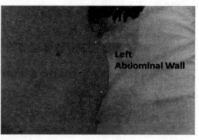

An important stabilizer of the back is the transversus abdominus. This muscle was likely cut through to get at the kidney, resulting in the muscle weakness you see above on the left side (inability to hold in the abdominal contents).

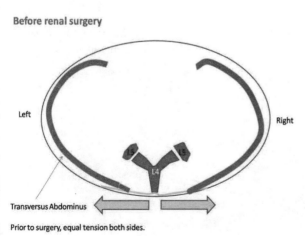

Before renal surgery

Left

Right

Transversus Abdominus

Prior to surgery, equal tension both sides.

Putting all of this together into the Ortho 2.0 triangle results in the following analysis. The transversus abdominus is a muscle that's the deepest of the abdominal wall. It attaches to the thoracodorsal fascia,and pulling on this muscle on both sides helps to allow the buoyancy of the abdominal contents to assist in offloading the weight of the upper body by literally floating it on the abdominal contents. <u>It's also a major low-back stabilizer all by itself</u>. The picture to the left shows that it attaches to fascia that then attaches to the back of the vertebra on both sides (spinous

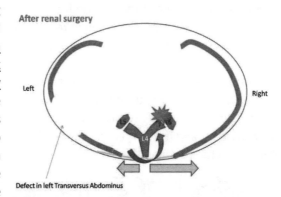

After renal surgery

Defect in left Transversus Abdominus

After surgery, poor pull from left TA causes slight left rotation of L4 vertebra causes right inferior articular process to move anterior.

process). The axial view ("saw"-you-in-half view) shows that if the pull is equal on both sides, this helps to keep the vertebra straight. However, if we cut one side of the transversus abdominus muscle (for example to get to a damaged kidney), the forces on the vertebra will be unequal, causing it to have a slight tendency to rotate (in this case to the left). The forces on the right facet joint will increase, causing more wear-and-tear forces on that side.

Below is an actual axial MRI image which shows the abnormal pull to the right by the transversus abdominus muscles (orange

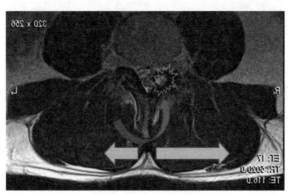

After renal surgery

arrows) causing extra force on the right facet joint (yellow star). This is where the facet cyst is located.

So, in summary, we believe that the damage to the ligaments in the back (supraspinous and interspinous ligaments) as well as this abnormal pull of one transversus abdominus over the other have caused the facet joints to wear out. Their response on the right (the side where we would predict the most force) is to swell to try and keep up with the wear and tear. This led to a facet cyst and then ultimately pressure on the spinal nerve. This complex example illustrates the importance of piecing together all of the parts and pieces of what caused the musculoskeletal system to fail. Many times, treating patients with musculoskeletal problems is as simple as a quick fix (in this case popping a facet cyst with a facet injection); other times it takes considerably more analysis.

Case 6: Pain Generator Gerry

Gerry is a middle-aged man who had a midfoot fusion that caused severe lateral ankle pain and grinding. A surgeon took an X-ray that showed arthritis at the talotibial joint and decided to replace that part of his ankle. This caused more severe lateral ankle pain and grinding. What went wrong?

Regrettably, the association between arthritis on X-ray and pain is pretty weak. Time and time again, research studies show that patients with arthritis or degenerative joints on X-ray are often asymptomatic. We have published on this issue in the low back, and the more recent discovery that 60% of knee meniscus tears don't cause pain has been blogged on in the past. There is also a study showing that pain causes arthritis, and not the other way around. This means that irritated nerves in the joint and presumably in the spine dump bad chemicals in the joint, which ultimately degrades the joint. So, with all of this data showing that we shouldn't rely on X-rays or MRIs to predict where pain is coming from, why do we see physicians performing surgery based solely on what they see on patient imaging? In this patient's case, an X-ray showing degeneration of her tibiotalar joint led to that joint being replaced. The pain got worse. Why?

Let's start with the concept of fusion. A fusion is where the surgeon places hardware (screws and plates) to make a solid structure. Bone is also usually placed in the area to literally grow the two joint surfaces into a solid mass of bone, further freezing motion. The concept began with surgeons treating bony multitrauma. This was a great advance that allowed surgeons to artificially fix a fracture through surgery with screws and plates and allowed the patient much more activity than placing him or her in a cast and in traction. This has been applied to degenerated joints more recently. The theory is that if the joint hurts, fusion will prevent motion in the joint, which will ultimately freeze its motion and eliminate the pain.

The problem with fusion is that all joints are connected. Fuse one joint and the motion that should be carried by that joint gets thrown to the next joint in line. This force transfer from the fused joint to the next joint often causes arthritis at the next overloaded joint. The poor next joint in line just wasn't designed to take that kind of force.

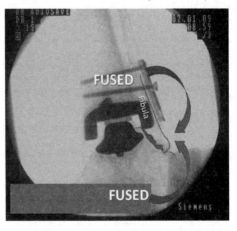

Let's look at this patient's fluoroscope image on the right. The fibula has been marked and the bottom part of it outlined. The first joints to be fused in the midfoot (the bottom area marked as "FUSED") caused those forces to be distributed to the joint between the bottom of the fibula (represented by the red arrow going up). This caused the joint between the end of the fibula and the rest of the foot (marked in red at the end of the fibula) to become overloaded and chronically painful. It likely also caused the other joint up the chain (the tibiotalar or one that was eventually replaced) to become degenerative. However, the catch was that the degenerated tibiotalar joint wasn't causing pain. So, when that joint was replaced (the bell-shaped dark-colored hardware and the downward-facing C-shaped hardware above that) the surgeon also placed the screws to fuse the fibula to the tibia (the area marked as "FUSED" where the screws are located). This then caused more overload of the joint below (the red arrow going down). This made the pain worse, as this was the painful joint to begin with (not the joint that was replaced). In the end, both the area below the painful joint and above that joint were fused, causing extra forces from above and below to be relayed into the painful joint. The result: more pain.

Could this have been prevented? Yes! The way to prevent this was to perform diagnostic numbing injections under X-ray to see which joint was causing pain. In the end, it would have been determined that the tibiotalar joint wasn't causing much pain (and, therefore, did not need to be replaced), and the joint between the end of the fibula and the rest of the ankle was causing pain. How do I know this? A numbing injection of this joint at the end of the fibula eliminated her severe pain with walking.

The take-home message? Big surgeries in the ankle and elsewhere can have big consequences that are many times irreversible. One should always take care to first diagnose where the pain is coming from before undergoing big surgeries. If needed, this includes diagnostic numbing injections. The same should hold true for any patient considering a joint replacement. Just because the joint looks bad on X-ray or MRI doesn't mean it's necessarily causing pain!

Appendix A—Regenexx in Healthcare

The *Regenexx Orthopedic Cost-Reduction Strategy* is a program for self-funded employers to address the rising costs of musculoskeletal care. Currently available to over seven million people across the United States, this program can be easily added to your insurance plan—and offers employees a nonsurgical approach to address their orthopedic pain without the need for invasive surgery.

Orthopedic issues such as osteoarthritis, torn or damaged ligaments and tendons, and various spinal injuries are the most prevalent reasons for doctor visits each year, the cost of these orthopedic injuries exceeding every other healthcare spend category (1)(2). Musculoskeletal (MSK) costs account for 15-30% of overall annual benefit expenses for self-funded employers, with the five-year average across all employers at 20% (3). The cost to treat major musculoskeletal issues—which often includes long-term pain management *and* disability—outpaces treatment costs for cancer, heart disease, and even diabetes (3).

Sadly, these costs are passed on to the consumer, increasing personal debt and causing many to delay the care they need today only to make their injury more difficult to manage tomorrow.

As described in this book, *Interventional Orthopedics* serves as a new step in the continuum of orthopedic care that can treat as many as 70% of structural problems without the need for invasive and costly surgeries*, and at significantly reduced cost.

And again, the *Regenexx Orthopedic Cost-Reduction Strategy* for self-funded employers can be easily added to health benefit plans, providing employees access to these procedures with coverage from the plan.

The Regenexx approach reduces the need for many elective orthopedic surgeries, providing significant cost-savings compared to the current orthopedic care continuum.

If you work for a company with roughly 200 or more employees, chances are they are self-funded. Please discuss the cost-saving strategy with your Human Resources or Benefits Department and have them contact Regenexx directly to see if our strategy can work for your company.

www.regenexxcorporate.com

References

1. https://www.mayoclinicproceedings.org/article/S0025-6196%2812%2901036-1/abstract
2. https://www.ribgh.org/documents/resources/Leading_Drivers_of_Employer_Healthcare_Spending_Growth.pdf
3. https://www.cnbc.com/2019/08/13/employee-health-benefits-costs-expected-to-rise-5percent-in-2020-new-survey-says.html

* This applies only to elective orthopedic surgery without fracture-related care or acute trauma.

Appendix B—Worksheets

These begin on the next page.

Regenexx Symmetry Test

Please fill out where you have tightness or pain by recording the letters on the figure that correspond to your problem areas. For example, in Step 1, if you have pain in the right shoulder with this stretch, you would place "A" in the blank for "Pain at___".

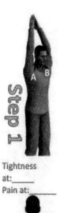

Step 1

Tightness at:_____
Pain at:_____

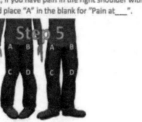

Step 5

Tightness at:_____ Pain at:_____

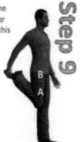

Step 9

Tightness at:_____
Pain at:_____

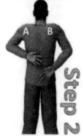

Step 2

Tightness at:_____
Pain at:_____

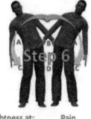

Step 6

Tightness at:_____ Pain at:_____

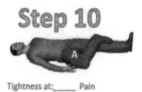

Step 10

Tightness at:_____ Pain at:_____

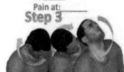

Step 3

Tightness at:_____ Pain at:_____

Step 7

Tightness at:_____ Pain at:_____

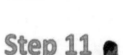
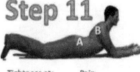
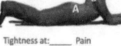

Step 11

Tightness at:_____ Pain at:_____

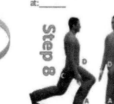

Step 4

Tightness at:_____ Pain at:_____

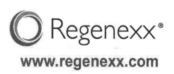

Step 8

Tightness at:_____ Pain at:_____

Regenexx®
www.regenexx.com

Write down your time:
___/20 seconds

Lie face down with your head off the end of a table or a firm bed as shown in A. Make sure your chest is stable and hold your head straight as shown in B. Time your endurance. When your head begins to fall downward or extend due to fatigue (as shown in C and D), the clock stops.

Write down your time:
Men:___sec/38
Women:__sec/29

Tuck chin and lift head about 2-3 inches and time. If any loss of height or chin tuck occurs, then stop timing. Normal is 38 sec for men and 29 sec for women.

___3-No difference between with and without the head hold
___2-Noticeable difference with arms all the way up
___1-Noticeable difference with arms above shoulder but not all the way up
___0-Can't get your arms over shoulder height

Lift arms above head all the way. Then have someone hold head firmly and retest. Fail if it's easier to lift the arms with head hold.

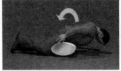

Write down your time:
Men:___sec/208
Women:__sec/124

Make sure your head/neck are flexed!

Lie on your stomach on a stiff pillow and extend your back so that your chest is off the floor and hold. Time how long you can hold this position.

___3-Able to do 30 reps easily w/o pain
___2-Much effort to get to 30 reps or pain with same
___1-Unable to finish 30 reps due to fatigue or pain
___0-Can't perform at all

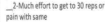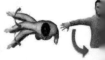

With arm out to the side with the **thumb down**, move the hand completely down and up in the three planes noted. Pass is at least 10 reps slowly (30 up-down movements.

Write down your time:
Right:___sec/10
Left:__sec/10

The clock stops when you lose any stability or look like the picture on the right!

Stand and balance on one leg and then perform a single leg deep knee bend. Hold for 10 seconds.

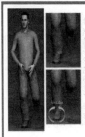

Stand on one leg as shown and try to balance while holding the ankle steady. Record the number of stable seconds for each side. The clock stops when your feel the wobble.

Write down your time:
Right:___sec/10
Left:__sec/10

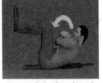

Write down your time:
Men:___sec/182
Women:__sec/85

Make sure your head/neck are flexed!

Lie on your back with your hips and knees both at 90 degrees and lift your torso off the ground. Time how long you can hold this position.

STABILITY

Self Assessment She[et]

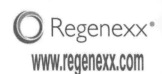

O Regenexx®
www.regenexx.com

About the Author

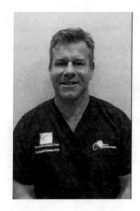

Christopher J. Centeno, MD, is a specialist in regenerative medicine and the new field of interventional orthopedics. He is board certified in physical medicine/rehabilitation and in pain management through the American Board of Anesthesia.

Dr. Centeno is one of the few physicians in the world with extensive experience in the culture expansion of and clinical use of adult stem cells to treat orthopedic injuries. He is a founding member of the International Cellular Medicine Society. His clinic incorporates a variety of pain management techniques, and he treats patients from all over the United States and the world who travel to Colorado to undergo innovative, nonsurgical treatments. Dr. Centeno's clinical practice in Colorado (The Centeno-Schultz Clinic) has a state-of-the-art cell biology research lab, a bioengineering department, and a clinical research arm.

Dr. Centeno has chaired multiple international research-based conferences. He also maintains an active research-based practice, with multiple publications listed in the U.S. National Library of Medicine. Dr. Centeno has also served as editor in chief of a medical research journal dedicated to traumatic injury. He has lectured all over the world on regenerative therapies, including at the Vatican in Rome.

Dr. Centeno trained at the Baylor College of Medicine, Texas Medical Center, and the Institute for Rehabilitation Research. He hails from both Florida and New York and currently resides in Boulder, Colorado, with his wife and three children.

Resources

Youtube Channel: Regenexx - https://www.youtube.com/user/Regenexx/videos

Ebooks: https://regenexx.com/resources/ebooks/

Find a Provider: https://regenexx.com/clinics/

Regenexx Blog: https://regenexx.com/blog/

Supplements: https://store.regenexx.com/

Other Books by Regenexx

Nutrition 2.0:
Guide to Eating and Living to Achieve a Higher Quality of Life Now and into Your Golden Years

By: Dr. John Pitts

Orthopedics 2.0:
How Regenerative Medicine and Interventional Orthopedics will Change Everything

By: Dr. Chistopher J. Centeno

Regenexx ProActive:
The Regenerative Orthopedic Program Designed to Ensure Peak Performance Well Beyond Middle-Age

By: Dr. Christopher J. Centeno

The Knee Owner's Manual:
How to Avoid Game Changing Invasive Knee Surgeries and Stay Active as You Age

By: Dr. Christopher J. Centeno

The Spine Owner's Manual:
How to Avoid Back Pain and Life Altering Surgery

By: Dr. Christopher J. Centeno